LOW FODMAP
MENUS for
Irritable Bowel Syndrome

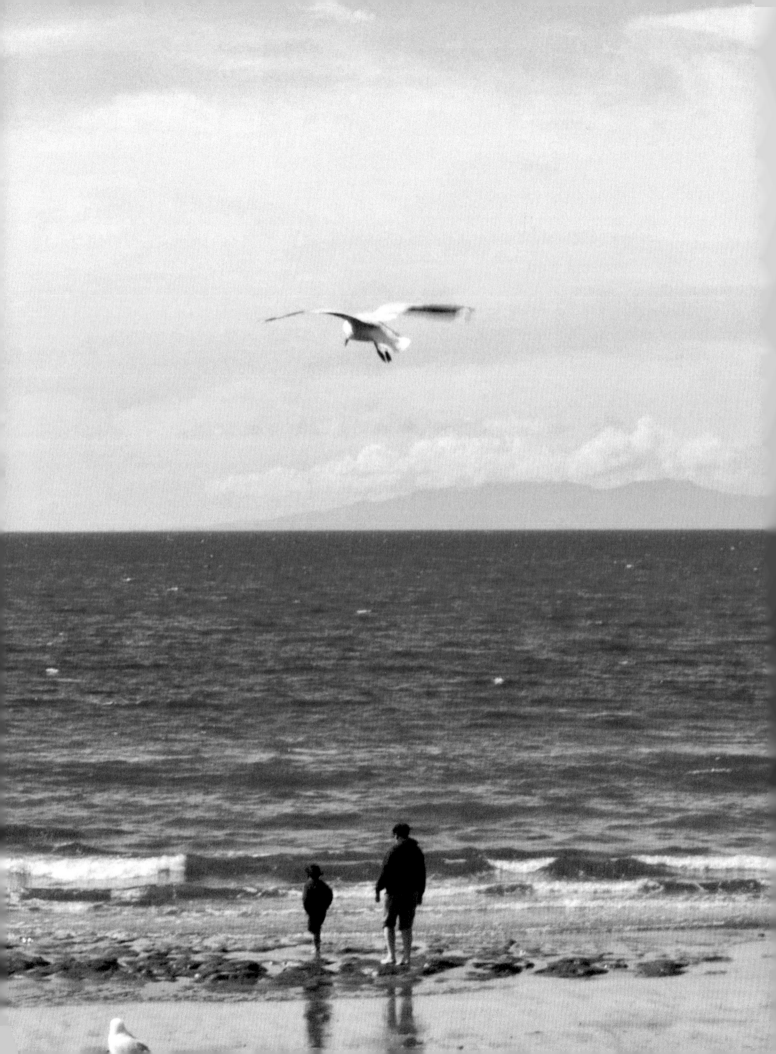

LOW FODMAP
MENUS for
Irritable Bowel Syndrome

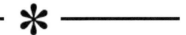

SUZANNE PERAZZINI

CREATOR OF *STRANDS OF MY LIFE*

photography & recipes by Suzanne Perazzini

LOW FODMAP
MENUS for
Irritable Bowel Syndrome

Written by: Suzanne Perazzini
Produced by: Suzanne Perazzini

www.strandsofmylife.com
suzanne.perazzini@orcon.net.nz

© 2014

COPYRIGHT

Design, Art Direction, Edited and Produced by Suzanne Perazzini

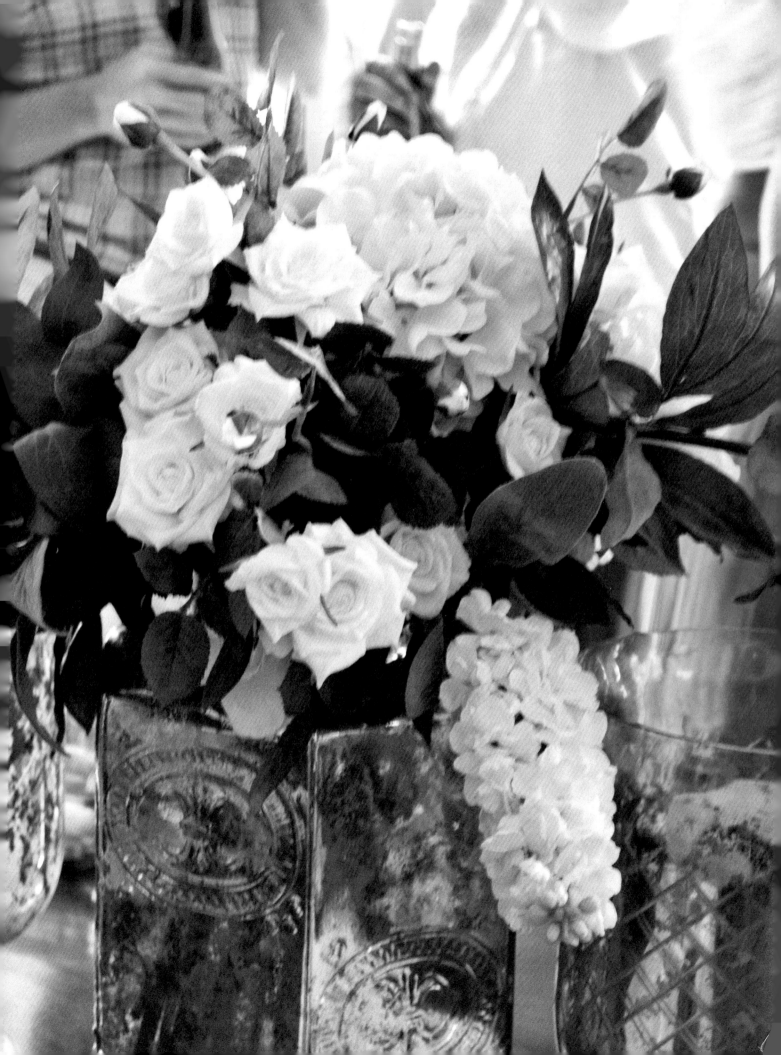

Contents

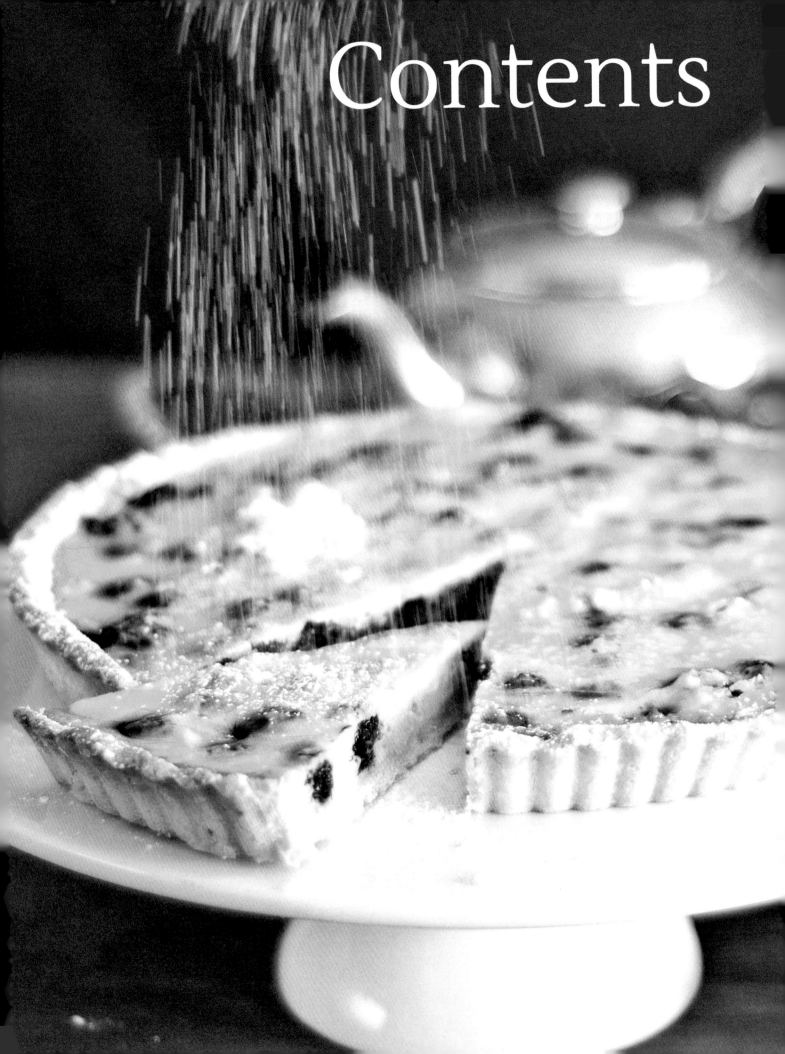

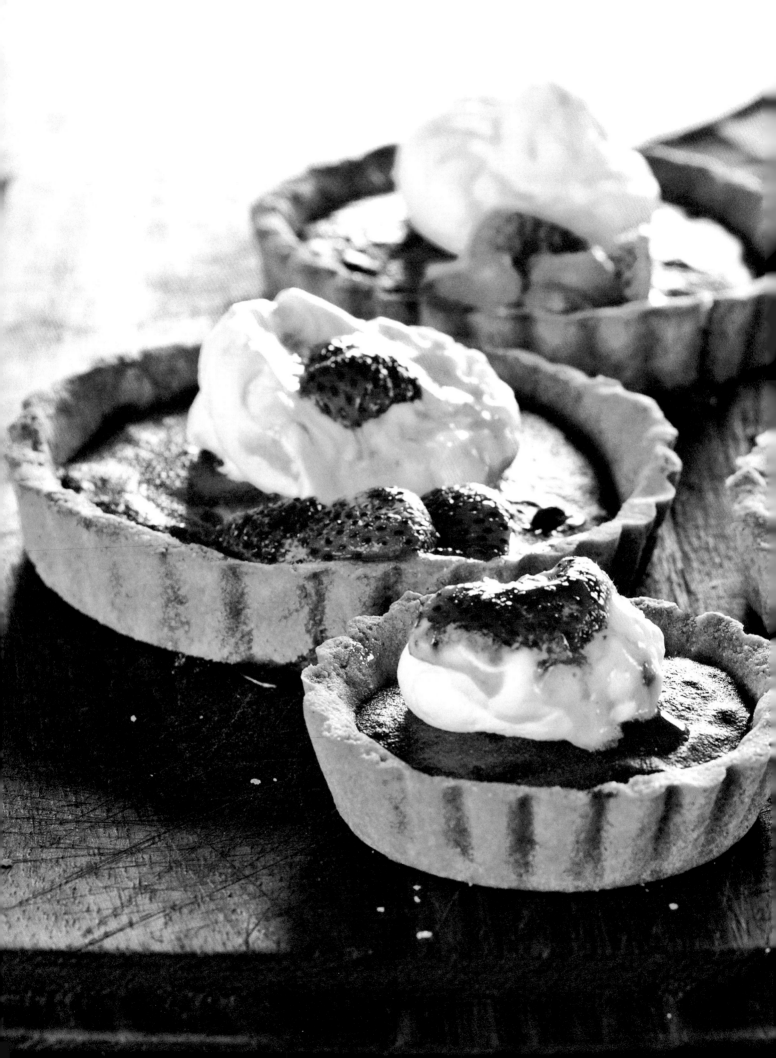

Introduction

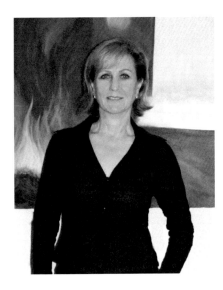

My name is Suzanne Perazzini and I am a super organized perfectionist who is a lover of travelling, reading, writing, photography and cooking. I live with my Italian husband and 23-year-old son in New Zealand in a house overlooking the Pacific Ocean.

I have suffered from digestive issues all my life. Through the years, I approached numerous doctors with my symptoms only to be told that I had irritable bowel syndrome and to eat more fibre, whole grains, fruit and vegetables. Each time I diligently went away and obeyed their instructions and felt worse than ever. They say that the definition of insanity is doing the same thing over and over and expecting a different result. I guess I was insane. For years!

Two years ago, I started my blog, Strands of My Life, as a way of exploring food and the effect it had on me. I tried various different diets and one day I Googled the heck out of my symptoms for the zillionth time, and the low FODMAP diet came onto my radar, and I realised I had seen it mentioned before but had glossed over it. I found an article that described the symptoms of someone who was intolerant to FODMAPs and I had a light bulb moment. This person was describing me, right down to how 'healthy' food made them worse. I investigated further and fructose malabsorption was mentioned. I knew almost immediately that I had hit the bullseye. The puzzle pieces were falling into place. I read about the hydrogen breath test for fructose malabsorption and had soon booked myself in for one. The test was positive. I was put onto a nutritionist who specialized in the low FODMAP diet, and I started the elimination portion of it. The improvement was rapid and surprising and miraculous. Some days I thought I could dance on water.

Almost two years later, there are days when I think I am feeling so good that I can test the limits of this diet, but then the symptoms return and I remember what it used to be like. There are good days and bad days but far more good days, and I am so grateful I could kiss the internet for the knowledge and information that is on there. I now blog, not to find a solution to my own issues, but so I can help others like me who are suffering and have suffered all their lives. This intolerance is a strange and difficult one to isolate. I had tried eliminating so many types of food in the past with no relief but I had never thought of something as complex as this. For the healthiest foods to be the culprits is almost unthinkable, and I now know why the doctors' advice always made me worse.

I have written this cookbook to help out those of you who, like me, must stick to the low FODMAP diet but struggle to come up with meal ideas. Your guests will expect desserts but always have only a small portion yourself if you have a problem with fructose.

I am the creator of the Inspired Life Low Fodmap Coaching Program to help those who are struggling with their IBS and the diet. If you would like to learn more about the program, please fill in the form at this link and I will give you a call: www.strandsofmylife.com/inspiredlife/

I hope you enjoy making these recipes.

Best wishes,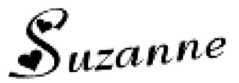

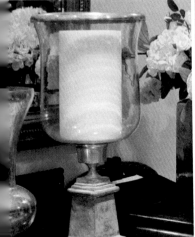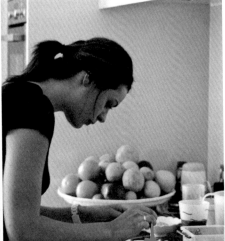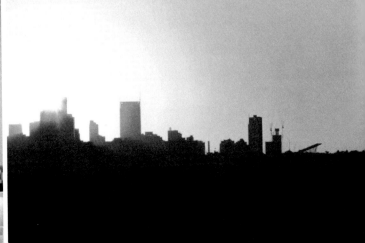

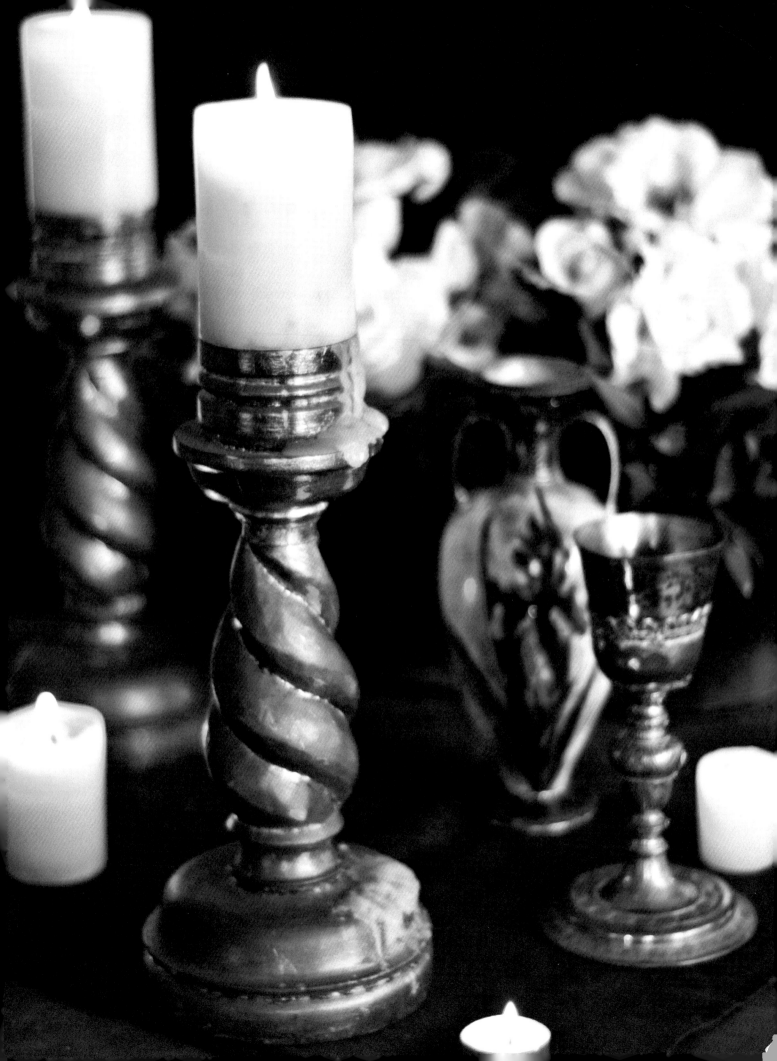

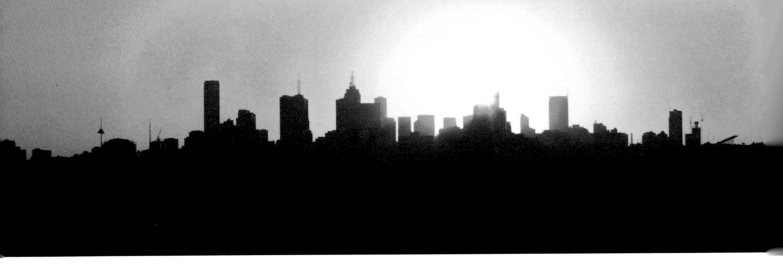

What are low FODMAPs?

FODMAP stands for Fermentable Oligo-saccharides, Disaccharides, Mono-saccharides and Polyols).

Fermentable:
The process through which gut bacteria break down undigested carbohydrate to produce gases (hydrogen, methane and carbon dioxide).

Oligo-saccharides:
Fructo-oligosaccarides (FOS) found in wheat, rye, onions and garlic.

Galacto-oligosaccharides (GOS):
Found in legumes/pulses.

Disaccharides:
Lactose found in milk, soft cheese, yoghurts etc.

Mono-saccharides:
Fructose (in excess of glucose) found in honey, many fruits and vegetables, high fructose corn syrups etc.

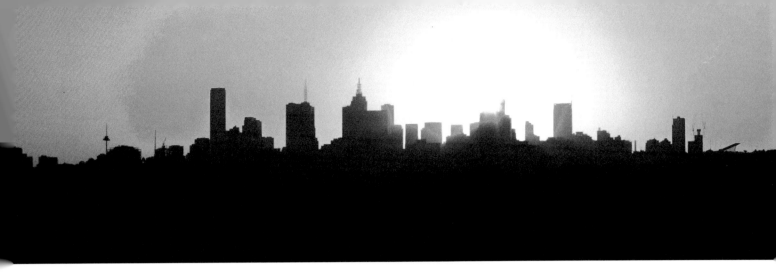

Polyols:

Sugar polyols (eg. sorbitol, mannitol) found in some fruit and vegetables and used as artificial sweeteners.

Anyone with irritable bowel syndrome has to try the low FODMAP elimination diet since FODMAPs are irritants of IBS. You can be tested for 2 of the 5 FODMAPs – fructose and lactose through a hydrogen test. But intolerance to the Oligo-saccharides and polyols can only be discovered through an elimination diet.

I had the hydrogen test which showed I absorbed fructose badly but that I was not lactose intolerant. Many who are intolerant to FODMAPs actually do fine with lactose so these recipes will include dairy, but it is relatively easy to replace it with lactose free alternatives. I have listed alternatives on page 19.

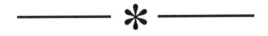

8 Signs of FODMAP Intolerance

No. 1. Food equals bloating

After you eat, does your stomach blow up and become taut as if it contains a football? If you poke it, is there very little give, only resistance? Your clothes become tight around the waist within a few minutes of eating. And it hurts.

No. 2. Healthy food seems to aggravate the problem

Many doctors have told you to eat more vegetables, fruit and whole grains so you can increase your fibre levels. But this makes you bloat worse than ever and gives you even more discomfort.

No. 3. You are lactose intolerant but...

The elimination of dairy hasn't solved all your problems. You know it has been a good move but why do you still get bloated and need to use the toilet more often than you would like?

No. 4. You can't identify the culprit(s)

Can you eat a particular food in the morning but the same food in the afternoon causes problems? Have you tried eliminating individual food groups without really improving things much? Are you totally confused about what foods really are the culprits even though you suspect some are not good for you? Maybe you have tried every food intolerance theory going but with little to no success? Food in general feels like your enemy.

No. 5. Doctors don't help

This relates to No.2. You have spoken to the doctor(s) many times over the years and tried desperately to explain the issues but they all give you the same advice (more fruit, veges and fibre), which only makes you feel worse. They use the irritable bowel syndrome diagnosis loosely which only manages to depress you.

No. 6. You have a love/hate relationship with the toilet

You have inconsistent toilet habits. Maybe you go four times a day because of diarrhoea, maybe you find it hard to go even once a day because of constipation. Maybe you often feel the urge to go but little happens in the toilet apart from the passing of wind. Is the feeling of incomplete evacuation of the bowels an issue?

No. 7. You feel better after going to the toilet

You rush to the toilet in pain and with a feeling of urgency. You may have diarrhoea or pass just a small motion but afterwards you feel relief from symptoms for several hours. But then you eat, and it comes back.

No. 8. Your digestive system rules your life

You make decisions based on the accessibility of a toilet. Going on holiday with other people with a shared bathroom is a nightmare. Travelling to out-of-the-way, exotic locales with limited toilet facilities is a dream tainted by major concerns. Accepting a job in a small firm with one shared toilet is probably not feasible.

These all could add up to intolerance to the FODMAPs in food. FODMAPS are present in almost all foods to some degree apart from a few like meat, chicken and fish. That is why you can't identify individual foods with ease. You can't stop eating everything else, so it becomes a matter of eliminating some foods and managing the rest. This is not simple but with help you can achieve it.

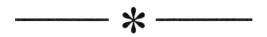

The 8 Symptoms of FODMAP Intolerance Explained

No. 1. Food equals bloating

FODMAPs like fructose should be absorbed through the lining of the small intestine, but when an individual has difficulty doing this, the fructose continues on down to the large intestine where it is treated as a foreign substance which causes the bacteria there to go to town. This results in bloating, diarrhoea or constipation, as well as flatulence and stomach pain as a result of muscle spasms. Intolerance to any or all of the FODMAPs will result in the same symptoms.

No. 2. Healthy food seems to aggravate the problem

For most people, including the 'experts', healthy food means fruit, vegetables, beans and whole grains (although the Paleo world would disagree with the last two). All three of those can be problematic for those with an intolerance to any or all of the FODMAPs. All fruits and vegetables contain fructose and many contain fructans and polyols, which can cause us problems. Some are lower in these substances than others and so can be tolerated in small helpings. Whole grains, in particular wheat, rye and barley, are high in fructans while beans contain fructans and GOS (galacto-oligosaccharides) – these are not at all good for us.

No. 3. You are lactose intolerant but...

Not all of those with FODMAP problems are lactose intolerant. In fact, I have no problem with dairy products, thank goodness. But it is logical to try eliminating them if you have digestive issues because lactose intolerance is well-known. This may or may not help depending on whether dairy is in fact an issue for you. I tried and it made no difference. But let's say you do see a difference but it hasn't solved the problem. That is because it is only one of the issues involved. Check out the other FODMAPS here. One or all of them could be the culprits.

No. 4. You can't identify the culprit(s)

I spent most of my adult life trying to find a solution to my bloating and other symptoms. I tried many elimination diets of the commonly known culprits like dairy and wheat, but none of them gave me an aha moment. I would then continue on with life and try to ignore the issue until something would prompt me to try again. Decades of frustration with no internet to Google for answers. No food blogs, dedicated to food intolerances. No information anywhere to help me. I envy those of you who have been born into this world governed by the internet. The answers are out there if you dig long and deep enough. No amount of digging was ever going to give me my answers before the internet was born because even the doctors didn't know about FODMAPs. That leads me on to the next point. But first I will briefly address the issue of the same food being a problem in the afternoon but not in the morning. FODMAPS accumulate in the body until they are released through going to the toilet. You will feel much better after a toilet visit and that's why. You have zeroed out the bad guys and can start accumulating again. So it's a delicate balancing act to keep the FODMAPs low enough in the digestive system to avoid the bloating and yet high enough to get the nutrition you need to survive. Not an easy one, but it can be done.

No. 5. Doctors don't help

I can't tell you how many doctors I have seen over my lifetime. In the last few years, I have changed doctors half a dozen times, always hoping that the next one would listen long enough to my symptoms to see that this was not a simple food intolerance. But they didn't. Right across the board they told me I had irritable bowel syndrome and to eat more fibre, fruit and vegetables. I would tell them that I already ate heaps of fibre, fruit and vegetables but usually by then my time would be up and they would give me a prescription for a fibre supplement. I did try some of the supplements but my symptoms always worsened. The problem is that FODMAP intolerance is not well-known and doctors do very little nutritional training, so are far from the experts we expect them to be where nutrition is concerned. And not one of them referred me to a nutritionist, who would be more up-to-date on the latest developments in their field. I did eventually go to one a few years back but she thought I had diverticulosis and gave me a diet for that. It helped a bit but not really.

No. 6. You have a love/hate relationship with the toilet

Most people with irritable bowel syndrome and/or a FODMAP problem either have diarrhoea or constipation. Diarrhoea is caused either by too much liquid entering the bowel or by food moving too fast through the bowel and there is no time for the normal drying out process to take place, or the drying out mechanism could be hindered by inflammation of the colon. Constipation is caused either by too little liquid or by too much drying-out because the contents of the bowel are moving too slowly or because you haven't gone to the toilet as soon as you felt the urge.

No. 7. You feel better after going to the toilet

This was explained above. When you zero out the FODMAPs, there is nothing to disturb your intestines so you feel great – for a while.

No. 8. Your digestive system rules your life

Of course this rules your life. I have always wondered what it would be like to not have to constantly think about this issue and to consider how it would impact on each of my decisions in life. I know now because I have it under control – finally. I seldom worry about toilets any longer but must always be aware of what goes into my mouth. If I suffer or not is now up to me. Not to fate.

Dairy Alternatives

My recipes use dairy because only 25% of those who have issues with FODMAPs are lactose intolerant, and it is easy to use alternatives. Remember that hard cheeses, butter and cream are mostly fine because they are the fat content of dairy and so have very little lactose in them. Here are a few alternatives to help you out if you are lactose intolerant:

Milk
Lactose-free milk, nut milks (be wary of too much almond milk though), rice milk, oat milk, coconut milk (1/2 cup only)

Butter (very low levels of lactose so a little won't hurt)
Vegan margarine (which has no hydrogenated oils)

Cheese (Hard cheeses have very low lactose)
Rice milk cheese, vegan cheeses (avoid those made from soya products)

Cream (very low levels of lactose so a little won't hurt)
Coconut cream (avoid using too much), nut creams (avoid using too much).

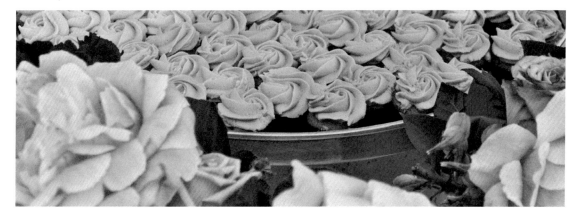

Foods you can and can't eat on the Low FODMAP Diet

We'll take each of the FODMAPs one by one and I'll tell you what to stay away from and what you can eat. These lists will be by no means complete but I will include the more common foods that most of us eat. See the note on page 23 to fully understand these lists.

FRUCTOSE

STAY AWAY FROM:

FRUIT

Apples, cherries, mangoes, pears, persimmom, watermelon

VEGETABLES

Sugar snap peas

SWEETENERS

Honey, high fructose corn syrup, fructose, fruit juice concentrate

YOU CAN EAT:

FRUIT

Apricots, avocados, bananas, blackberries, blueberries, boysenberries, grapefruit, grapes, kiwifruit, lemons, limes, mandarins, nectarines, oranges, passionfruit, peaches, pineapple, plums, raspberries, rhubarb, strawberries, tomatoes - all in moderation.

VEGETABLES

All except sugar snap peas.

SWEETENERS

Golden syrup, maple syrup, rice syrup, table sugar, cane sugar, icing sugar, brown sugar, raw sugar, glucose - all in moderation.

FRUCTANS

STAY AWAY FROM:
FRUIT
Nectarines, watermelon, persimmon, white peaches.

VEGETABLES
Artichokes, asparagus, beetroot, Brussels sprouts, cabbage, fennel, garlic, leeks, onions, peas, spring onions.

GRAINS & STARCHES
Wheat, rye and barley.

LEGUMES
Chickpeas, lentils and all legume beans.

NUTS
Pistachio, go easy on almonds

YOU CAN EAT:
FRUIT
All other fruits except those above - all in moderation.

VEGETABLES
Avocados, bok choy, broccoli, capsicums, carrots, cauliflower, celery, cucumber, ginger, green beans, lettuce, mushrooms, potatoes, pumpkin, spinach, sweet potatoes, tomatoes, zucchini.

GRAINS & STARCHES
Amaranth, arrowroot, buckwheat, maize, millet, oats, potato, quinoa, rice, sorghum, tapioca.

GALACTO-OLIGOSACCHARIDES

STAY AWAY FROM:
Chickpeas, lentils, dry beans like kidney, borlotti, haricot, pinto, navy, lima, soy, broad.

YOU CAN EAT:
There are none that you can eat.

LACTOSE

STAY AWAY FROM:
Animal milk – cow, sheep, goat, yoghurt, ice cream, cream cheese, cottage cheese.

YOU CAN EAT:
Lactose-free dairy products, hard and ripened cheeses, butter, cream (these are virtually lactose free.)

POLYOLS

STAY AWAY FROM:
FRUIT
Apples, apricots, blackberries, cherries, pears, peaches, plums, prunes, watermelon.

VEGETABLES

Avocados, cauliflower, mushrooms, snowpeas.

ADDITIVES

Sorbitol, mannitol, maltitol, xylitol (as in diet gums, lollies, dairy desserts etc.

YOU CAN EAT:

FRUIT

Bananas, blueberries, boysenberries, cranberries, grapefruit, grapes, kiwifruit, lemons, limes, mandarins, mangoes, oranges, passionfruit, pineapple, raspberries, rhubarb, strawberries - all in moderation.

VEGETABLES

All except those mentioned above.

ADDITIVES

Aspartame, saccharine, stevia (that's not to say you should use artificial sweeteners).

Note: What you will see above is that a food might be fine under one list but not under another. For example: blackberries are low in fructose but high in polyols. If you know you malabsorb fructose but are fine with polyols, then you can eat them. You have to cross-reference the lists to get the ultimate list that suits you.

Source: Food Intolerance management Plan by Dr Sue Shepherd and Dr Peter Gibson

BRUNCH

Feta & poached egg sandwich

Salmon & courgette stacks

Potato & cheese muffins

Banana & blueberry loaf

Serves 6

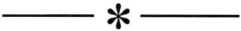

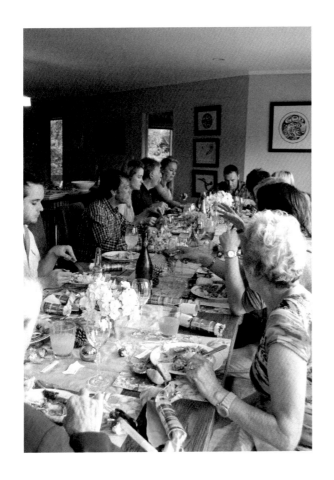

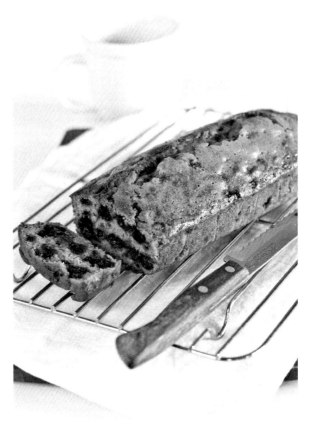

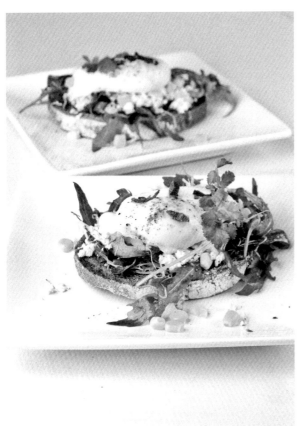

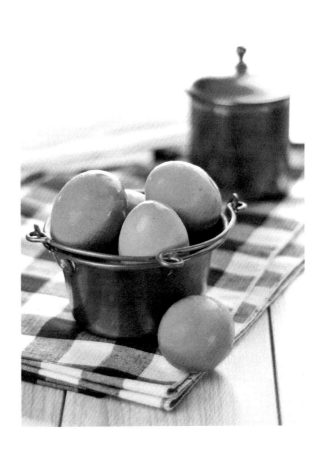

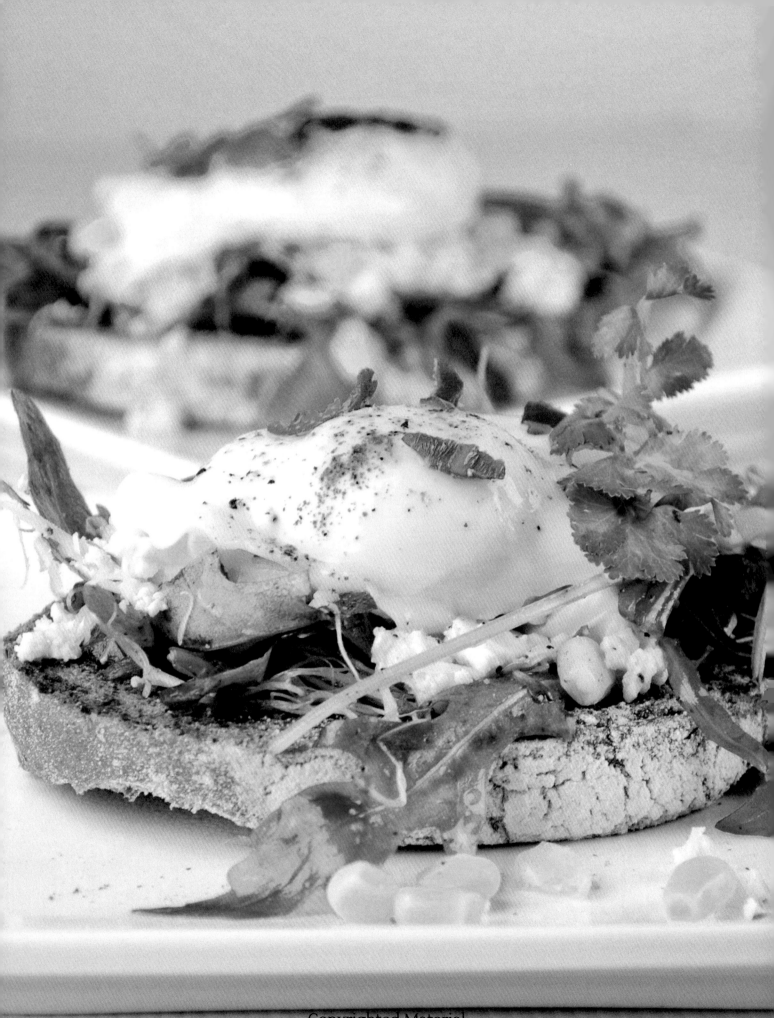

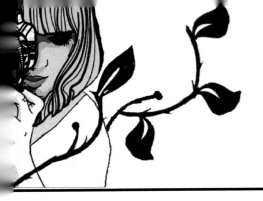

Feta & Poached Egg Sandwich

Slices of gluten-free bread (Page 75)

A packet of arugula

Alfalfa sprouts

Corn, cooked & scraped from the cob

(1/2 cob of corn is low Fodmap)

Olive oil

Lemon juice

Salt & pepper

Six eggs

150gms/5.3oz feta cheese

1 tbsp grated parmesan

A pinch of dried or 1 tsp fresh thyme

1 chilli - sliced finely

Paprika

1. Toast or grill the bread.

2. Crumble the feta and mix with the parmesan, thyme and a little lemon juice.

3. Dress the arugula and sprouts with oil, lemon juice, salt and pepper.

4. Poach the eggs.

5. Assemble the sandwiches with first the salad mix, then the cheese mix, then the corn and place the egg on top.

6. Season the egg and sprinkle with paprika and the red chillies.

Strands of My Life

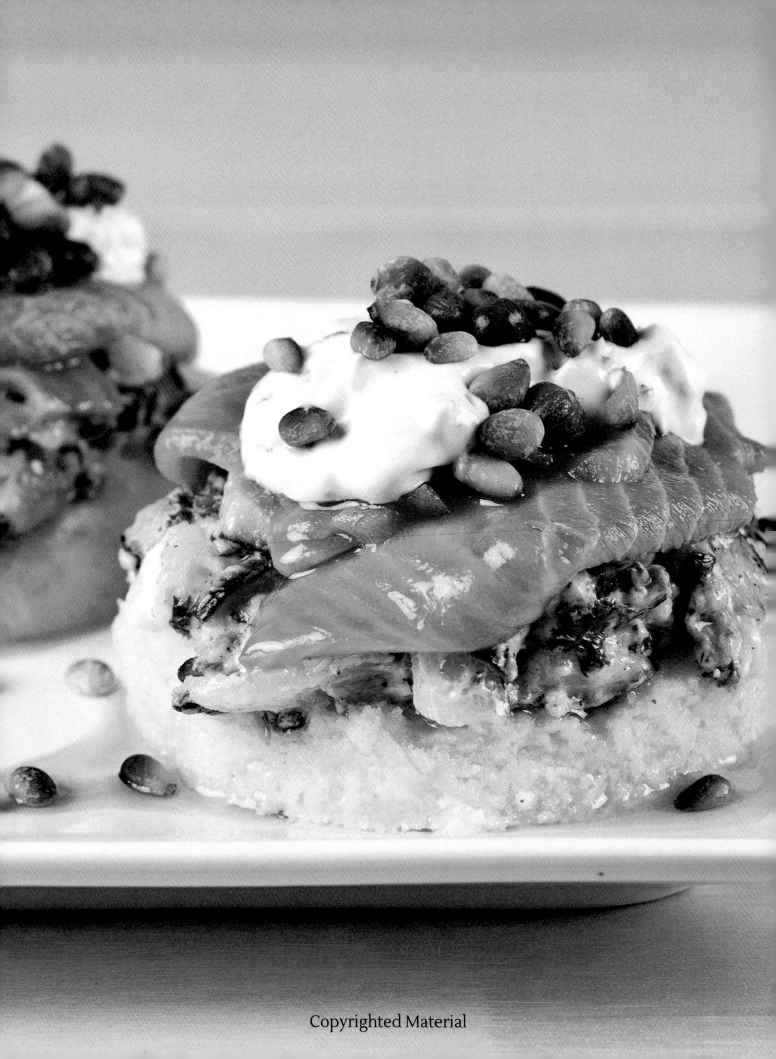

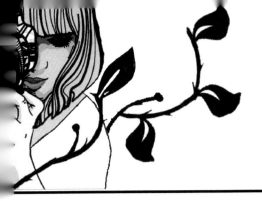

Salmon and Courgette Stacks

1 packet of Polenta

4-5 zucchini

1 tbsp cream cheese

Small bunch of Parsley

2 tsp rice bran oil

2 tsp garlic-infused olive oil

Salt & pepper

12 slices of smoked salmon

3 tbsp capers

3 tbsp pine nuts

6 tbsp sour cream

2 tsp lemon juice

Note: see page 19 for dairy alternatives

1. Chop up the zucchini and fry in the rice bran oil and garlic-infused olive oil until soft.

2. Add the cream cheese and season.

3. Finely chop half the parsley and add to the zucchini.

4. Cook the polenta according to the instructions on the packet.

5. Turn out onto a wooden board and flatten to about 1"/2.5cm thick.

6. Cut out rounds and place on a serving plate.

7. Place spoonfuls of the courgette mixture on top of the rounds.

8. Layer slices of salmon over the courgettes.

9. Mix the sour cream with the lemon juice, season and add the rest of the parsley.

10. Place a spoonful of the sauce on top of the salmon.

11. Sprinkle with capers.

12. Toast the pine nuts and sprinkle over as well.

Strands of My Life

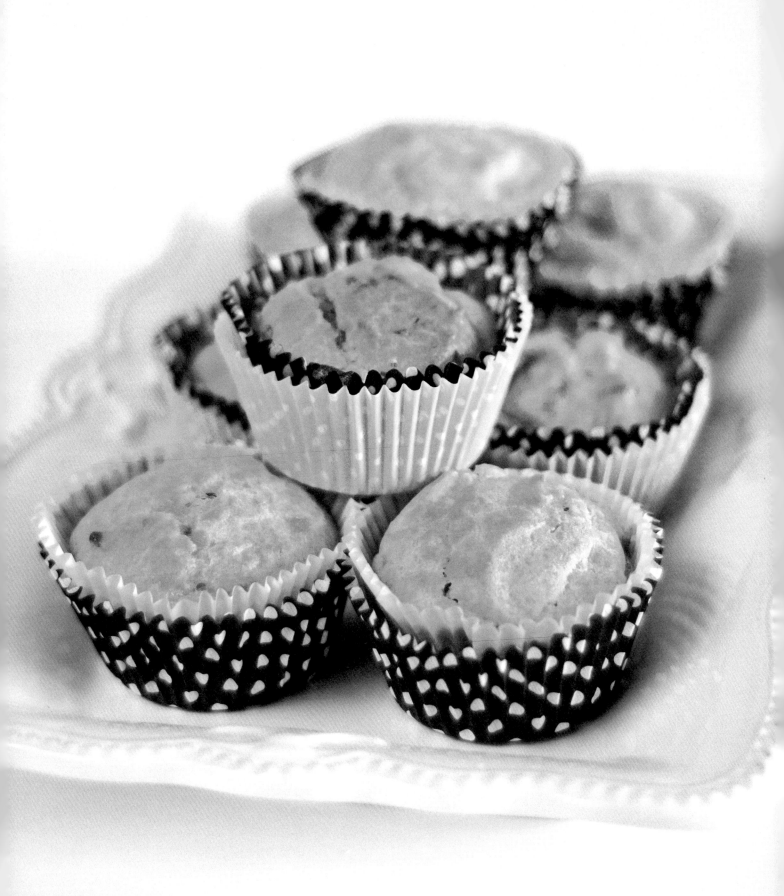

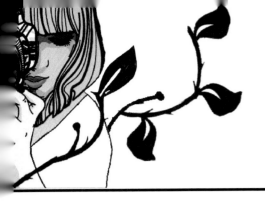

Potato & Cheese Muffins

250gms/8.8ozs cooked potato

1 cup water

1 cup coconut or rice bran oil

2 eggs

1.3 cups white rice flour

1/3 cup tapioca flour

1/3 cup potato starch

2 tsp baking powder

pinch of salt

1 tsp paprika

1/4 tsp black pepper

1 cup hard cheese

1. Heat oven to 180°C/350°F.

2. Place the cooked potato, water, eggs and oil in a food processor and blend well.

3. Sift the dry ingredients together.

4. Add the wet ingredients to the dry.

5. Stir in the grated cheese and mix well.

6. Place cupcake papers into a 12 capacity muffin tin.

7. Lightly spray them with coconut oil.

8. Spoon the mixture into the cupcake papers.

9. Bake for about 20 minutes.

10. Let cool a little and eat fresh.

Strands of My Life

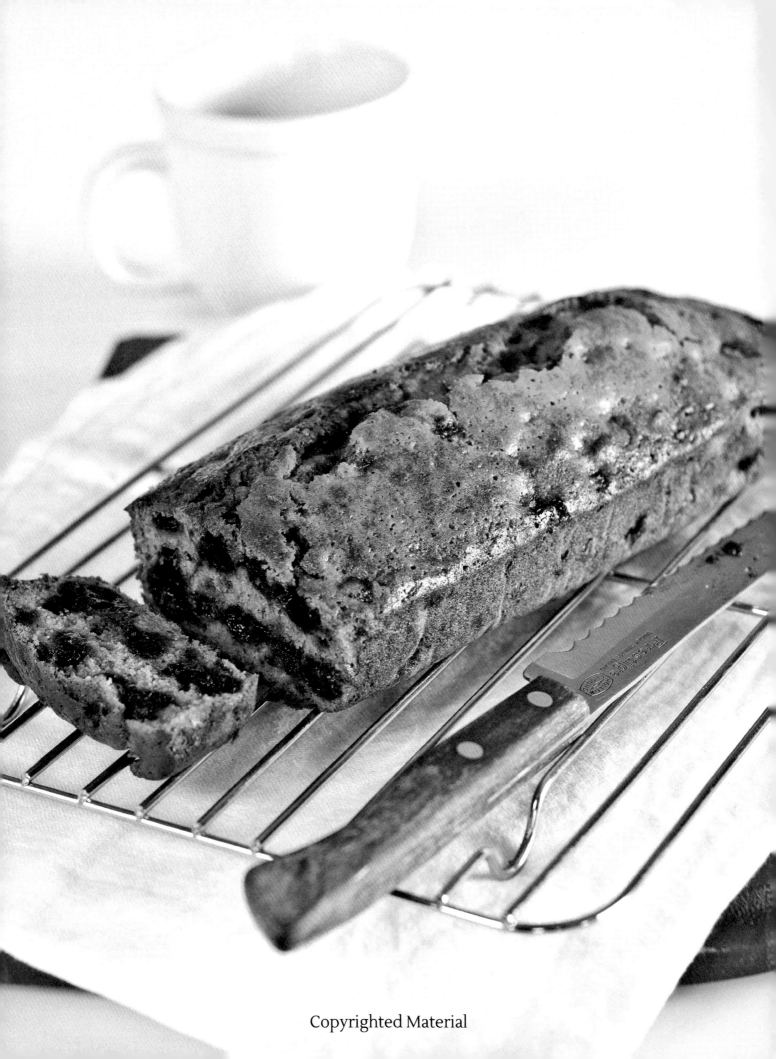

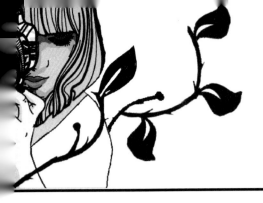

Banana & Blueberry Loaf

1 banana

1 medium potato boiled and mashed

57gms/2 oz melted unsalted butter

1 tsp vanilla essence

2 eggs

2 tbsp chia seeds

1/2 cup sugar

1/3 cup white rice flour

1/3 cup brown rice flour

1/4 cup tapioca flour

1/4 cup potato starch

1 tsp cinnamon

1 tsp baking powder

1/2 tsp baking soda

pinch of salt

1 cup blueberries (fresh or frozen)

1. Heat oven to 180°C/350°F.

2. In a food processor, blend the banana, potato, butter and vanilla.

3. Add the eggs and blend again.

4. Sift all the dry ingredients together.

5. Add the dry ingredients to the wet and mix well.

6. Add the blueberries and mix gently.

7. Pour the mixture into a lined loaf tin and bake for 1 hour.

8. Cool completely before slicing.

Strands of My Life

LADIES' LUNCH

Blinis with salmon & sour cream

Mediterranean pies

Greek salad

Trifle cakes

Serves 6

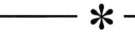

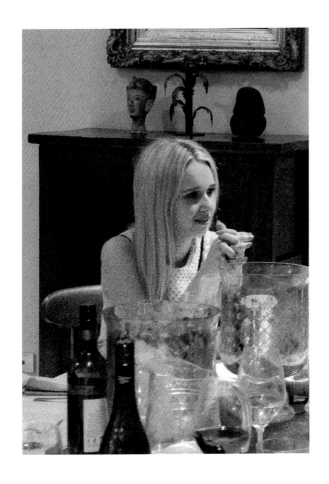
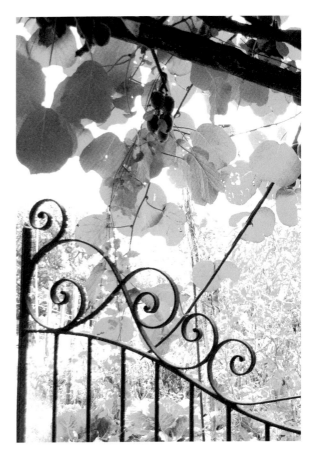
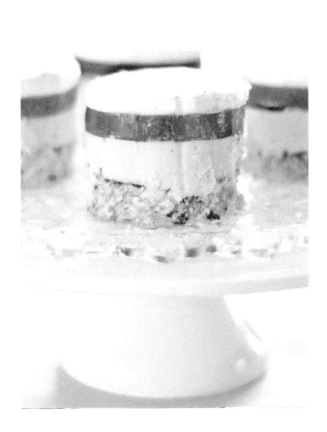
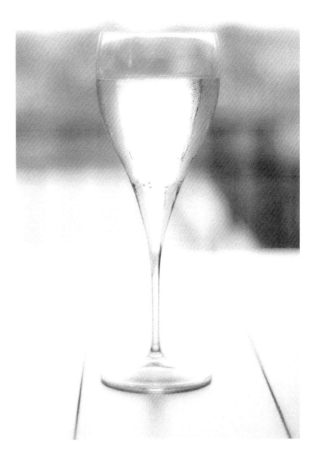

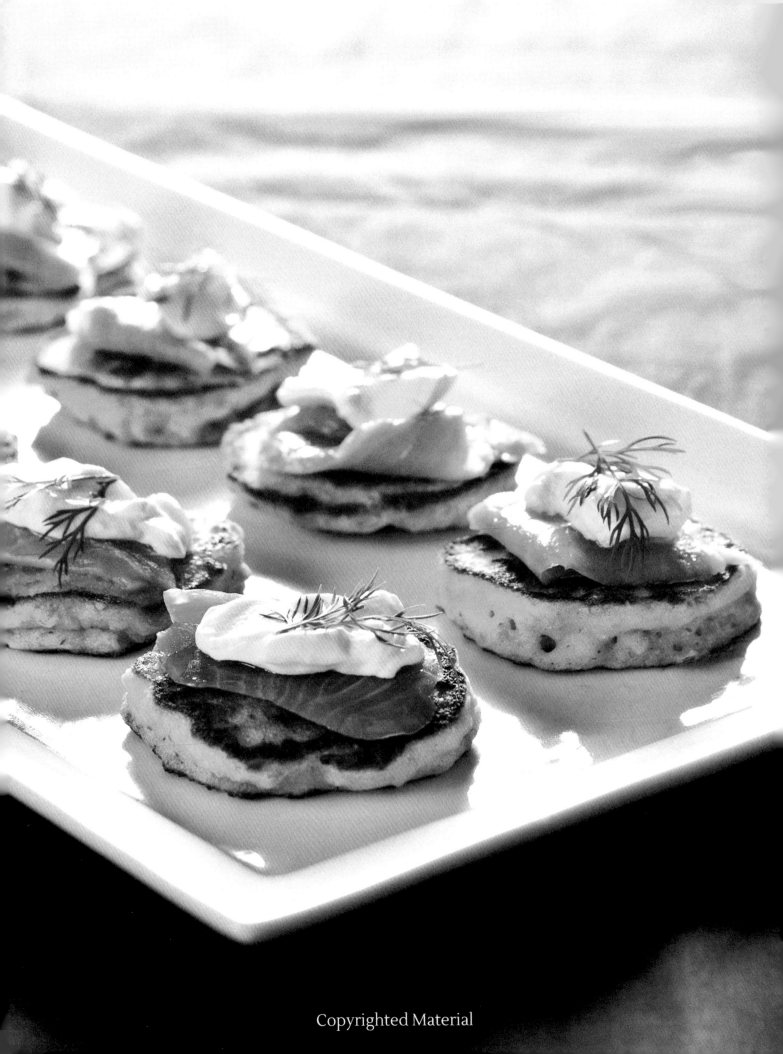

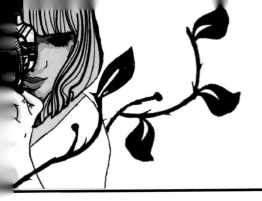

Blinis with Salmon & Sour Cream

For the blinis:

1 cup milk

½ cup of water

1 tbsp lemon juice

¼ cup of melted butter

3 eggs

1 cup oats

2/3 cup white rice flour

5 tbsp tapioca flour

6 tbsp potato starch

1 tsp baking powder

½ tsp baking soda

1 tsp cumin

Pinch of salt

For the topping:

Smoked salmon

Sour cream

Dill

Note: see page 19 for dairy alternatives

For the blinis:

1. Sift the flours, salt, baking powder, baking soda and cumin together.

2. Whisk together the wet ingredients.

3. Add the wet to the dry ingredients and blend well.

4. Place the mixture in the fridge for 10 mins.

5. Heat a frying pan and drop in a small knob of butter to melt.

6. Spoon in enough mixture to create a mini pancake of the size you want.

7. Repeat until the frying pan is filled.

8. When bubbles form all over the tops, flip them over.

9. When they are also browned on the other side, remove and place on a serving dish.

10. Repeat with the rest of the mixture.

For the topping:

11. Place portions of salmon doubled over on each blini.

12. Spoon over a dollop of sour cream on each slice of salmon.

13. Garnish with a small piece of dill.

Strands of My Life

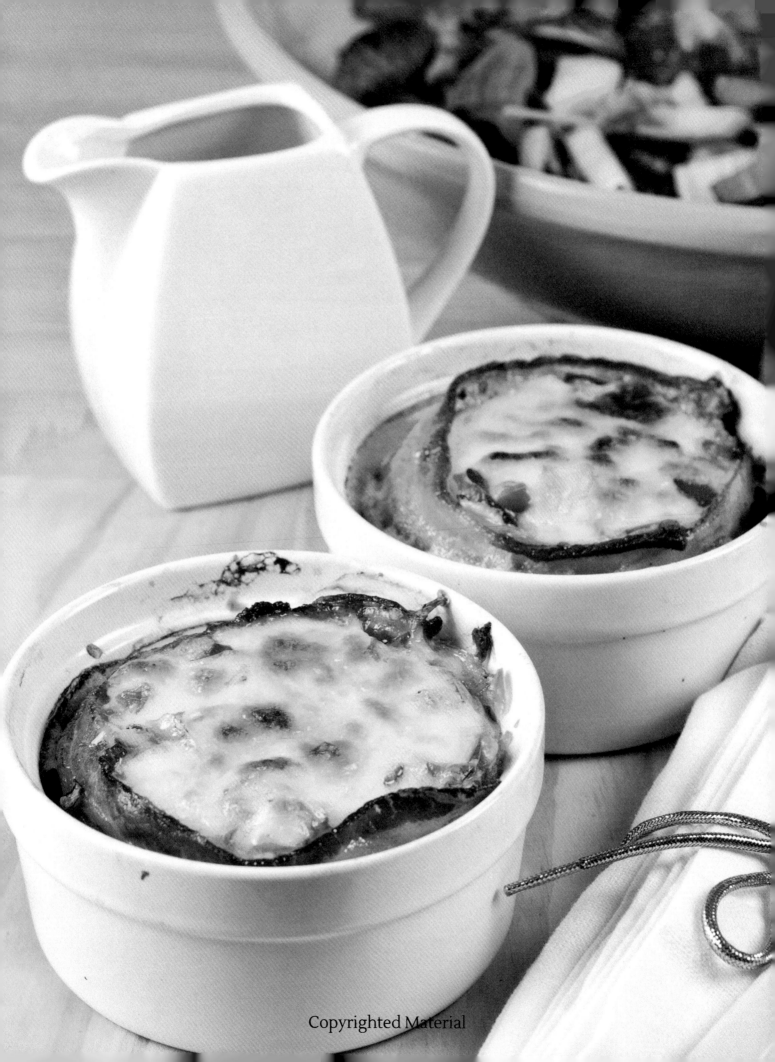

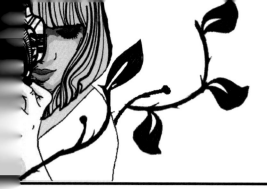

Mediterranean Pies

12 rashers of rindless bacon

2 zucchini, diced

2 red pepper, cored and diced

1 green pepper, cored and diced

1 large carrot, peeled and diced

6 eggs, beaten

1.5 cups grated mozzarella

Salt and pepper

1. Preheat oven to 180°C/350°F.

2. Line 6 small dishes with bacon.

3. Mix the chopped up vegetables in a bowl.

4. Spoon the mixture into the 6 dishes.

5. Beat the eggs and season.

6. Pour over the vegetables.

7. Sprinkle with mozzarella.

8. Bake for 20 – 25 minutes until the egg is set and the cheese browned.

Strands of My Life

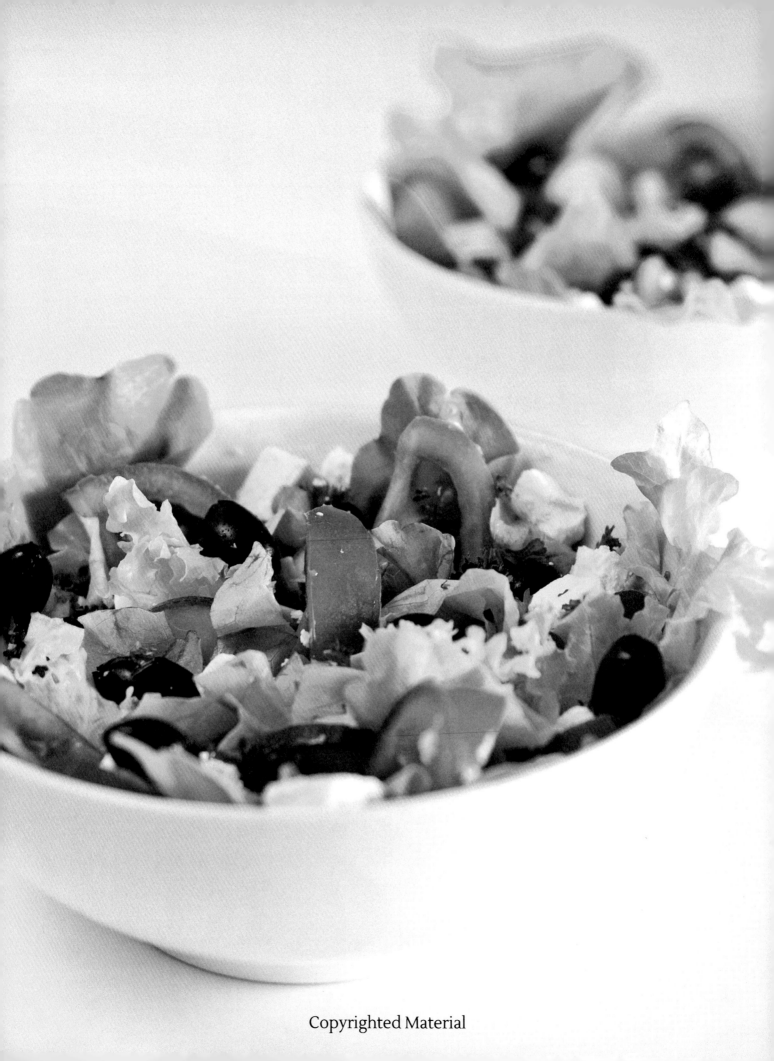

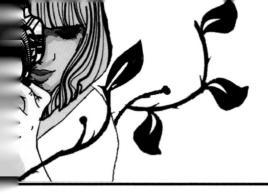

Greek Salad

For the salad:

300gms/7oz feta cheese

Lettuce

6 tomatoes, cut in wedges

2 zucchini

a small tub of pitted black olives

Chopped parsley

For the dressing:

1/3 cup olive oil

2 tsp garlic-infused olive oil

3 tbsp lemon juice

Salt and pepper

For the salad:

1. Cut the feta into small squares.

2. Slice up the zucchini.

3. Break the lettuce into pieces.

4. Place all the ingredients for the salad into a serving bowl.

For the dressing:

1. Place all ingredients into small jar and shake to combine well.

2. Pour over the salad just before serving and toss.

Strands of My Life

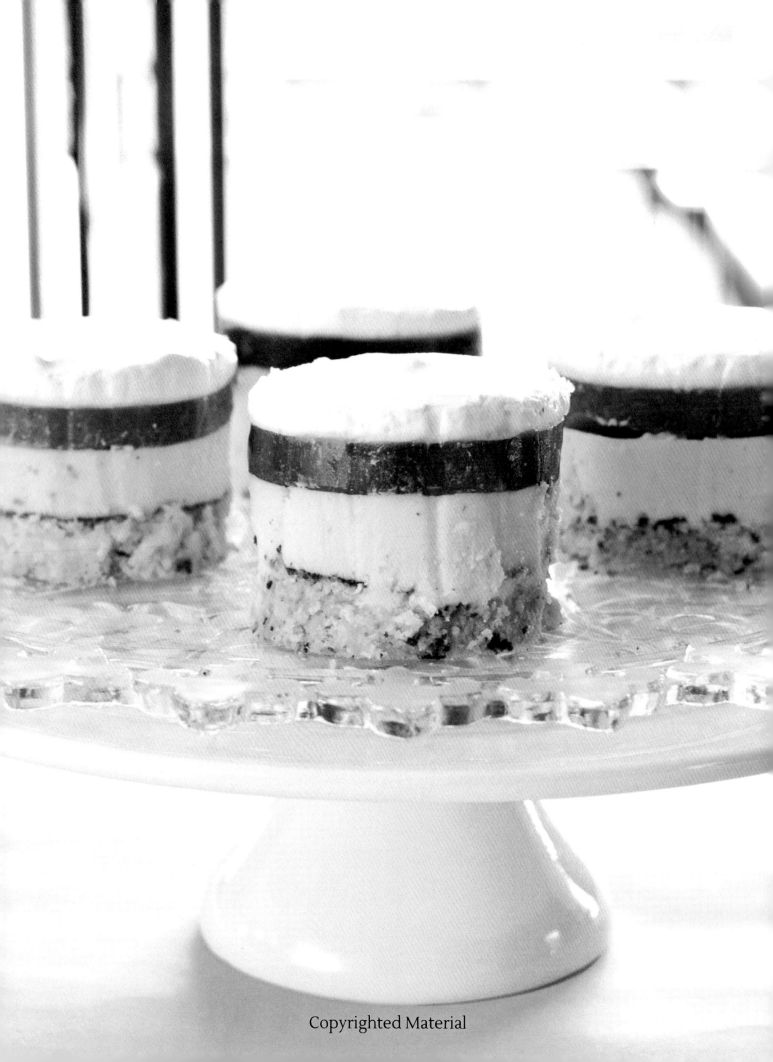

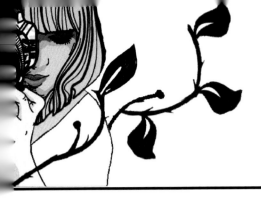

Trifle Cakes

For the base:

Use the cake recipe on page 61 without the strawberries

For the custard:

400mls/13.5oz cream

3 tbsp sugar

1/3 cup lemon juice

2 tbsp gelatin

1 tbsp tapioca flour

36 blueberries

For the jelly:

1/2 cup water

4.5 tsp gelatin

490 mls/16.5oz fresh orange juice, strained

6 tbsp caster sugar

1/2 cup your favourite liquor

For the marshmallow:

2 tbsp gelatin

4 tbsp water

1.5 cup caster sugar

1 cup water

1 tsp vanilla

Note: see page 19 for dairy alternatives

For the base:

1. Cut four rounds out of the cake and place in the base of six 3"/7.5cm moulds.

For the custard:

2. Bring the cream and sugar to the boil, add the juice and stir.
3. Dissolve the gelatine in 1tbsp hot water and whisk in.
4. Mix the tapioca flour in a little cold water and add.
5. Keep stirring until thick then take off the heat and let cool before pouring over the cake bases.
6. Place six blueberries spaced out on top of the custard and push them into it and place in the fridge to set completely.

For the jelly:

7. Place the water in a bowl and sprinkle over the gelatin.
8. Place the juice and sugar in a pan and heat until the sugar is dissolved and add the softened gelatin and simmer for 5 mins.
9. Remove from the heat, add the liquor and cool completely.
10. Pour over the set custard layer and place in the fridge.

For the marshmallow:

11. Sprinkle the gelatin over the first lot of water and let it absorb.
12. Place the sugar and the second lot of water in a saucepan and bring to the boil, stirring.
13. Boil, not stirring, for 15 mins. Add the gelatin and boil for 4 mins.
14. Cool to lukewarm and add the vanilla.
15. With egg beaters or a stand mixer, whisk until thick and white.Spoon onto the set jelly layer and place in the fridge to firm up.
16. Once set completely, carefully remove the moulds.

Strands of My Life

BEACH PICNIC LUNCH

Salmon & spinach quiche

Bacon pasta salad

Carrot cake

Creamy lemon tarts

Serves 6

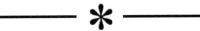

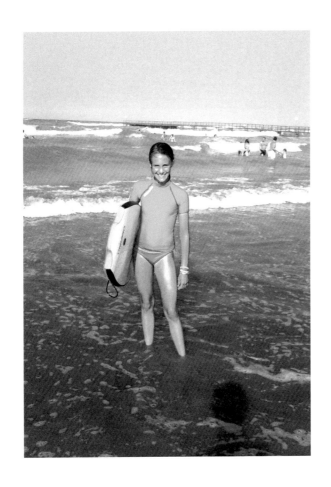

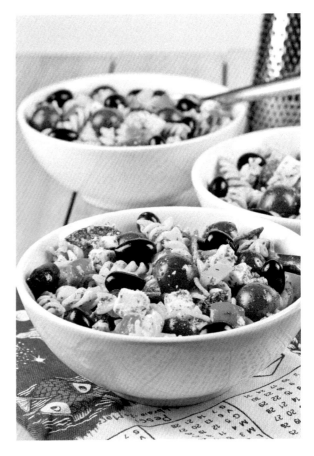

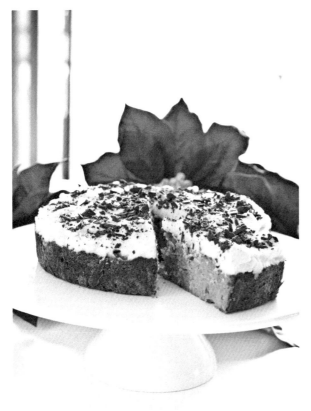

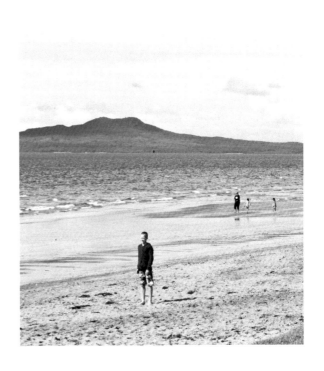

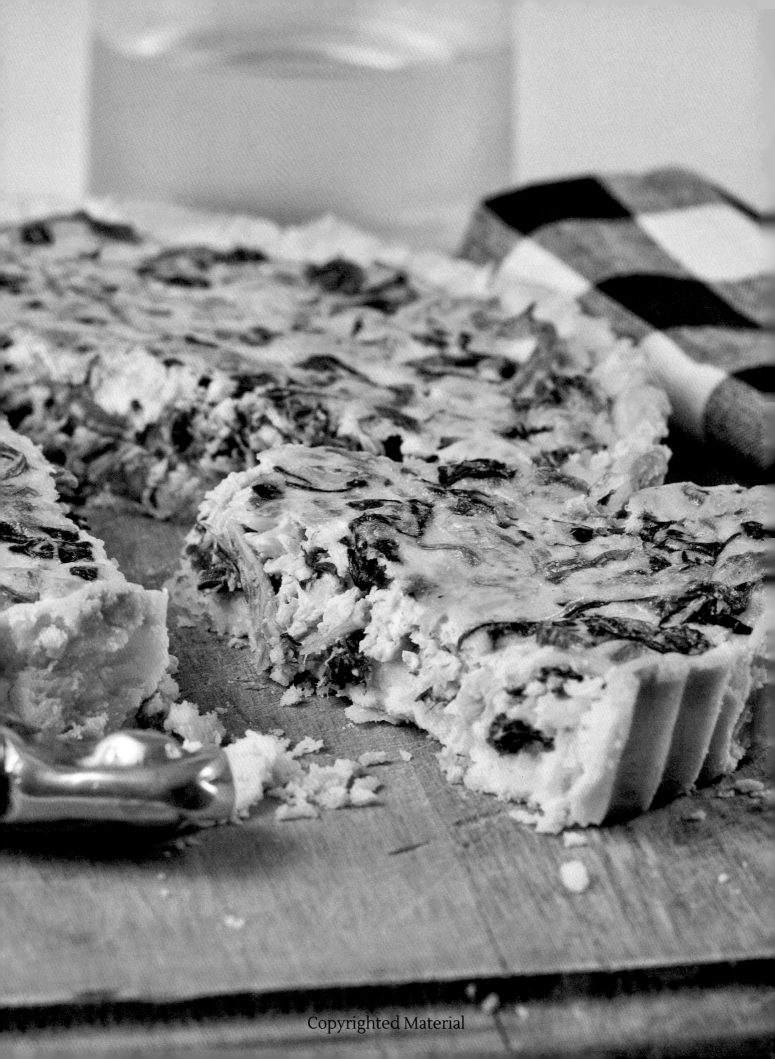

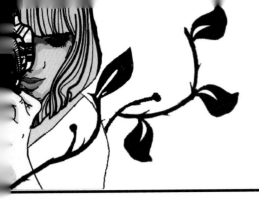

Salmon & Spinach Quiche

For the pastry:

133gms/4.7oz white rice flour

22gms/0.8oz tapioca flour

45gms/1.6oz potato starch

Pinch of salt

100gms/3.5oz butter

1 medium egg

For the filling:

1 good sized salmon fillet

A few slices of lemon

A few peppercorns

A pinch of salt

125g/4oz chopped spinach

200mls/7 fl. oz sour cream

2 eggs, beaten

Black pepper

Note: see page 19 for dairy alternatives

For the pastry:

1. Blend all the dry ingredients in a food processor.
2. Add the butter cut into small pieces to the food processor and process until fine crumbs form then add the egg and process until it forms a dough.
3. Remove from the processor and add a little more rice flour if it is too wet.
4. Press out into greased 23cm/9in quiche baking dish and place in the fridge for 30 minutes.
5. Heat the oven to 180°C/350°F.
6. Line the pie crust with baking paper and fill with baking beans.
7. Bake for 5 minutes, remove the beans and cook for 5 more minutes.

For the filling:

8. Poach the salmon in boiling water into which you have put the peppercorns, lemon and salt.
9. Once cooked (5-8 minutes), remove and dry with paper towels and flake into bite-sized pieces.
10. Place the salmon and all the other ingredients into a bowl and stir carefully.
11. Pile into the pastry case and bake for 25 minutes or until the filling is set.
12. Let stand for 10 minutes to firm up before cutting.

Strands of My Life

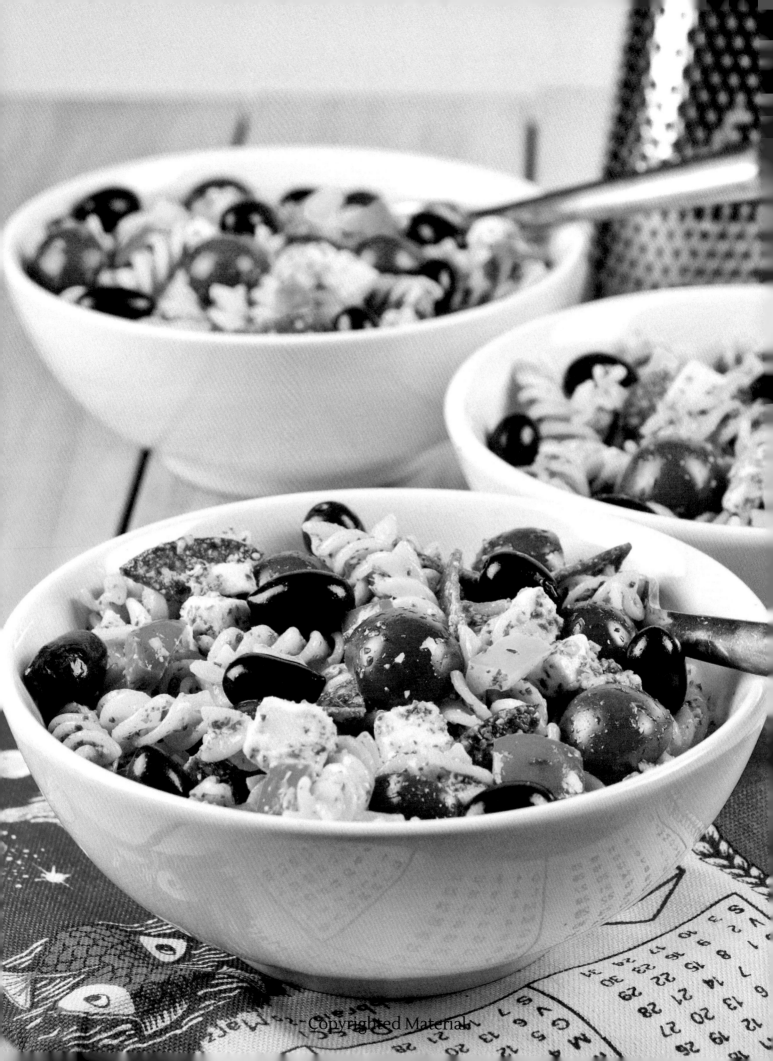

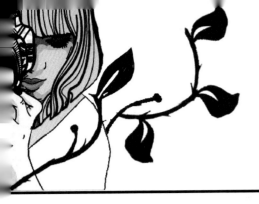

Bacon Pasta Salad

For the salad:

10 slices of bacon

400gms/14oz gluten-free pasta

A punnet of cherry tomatoes

A handful of black olives

1 yellow pepper

1 orange pepper

1 mozzarella

For the pesto:

A bunch of basil

2 tbsp pine nuts

40gms/1.4oz Parmesan

1 tbsp garlic-infused oil

1/2 cup olive oil

Salt & pepper

For the salad:

1. Cut the bacon into small squares and fry in a tiny bit of oil. Drain on absorbent paper.

2. Cook the pasta according to the packet instructions, drain well and toss through a little olive oil to keep it from sticking.

3. Dice the peppers.

4. Cut up the mozzarella into cubes,

5. Place all the ingredients in a serving bowl and toss through with the pesto sauce.

For the pesto:

6. Place everything except the oils in a food processor and process until well chopped.

7. Drizzle in the oil while the machine is running.

8. Adjust the seasoning.

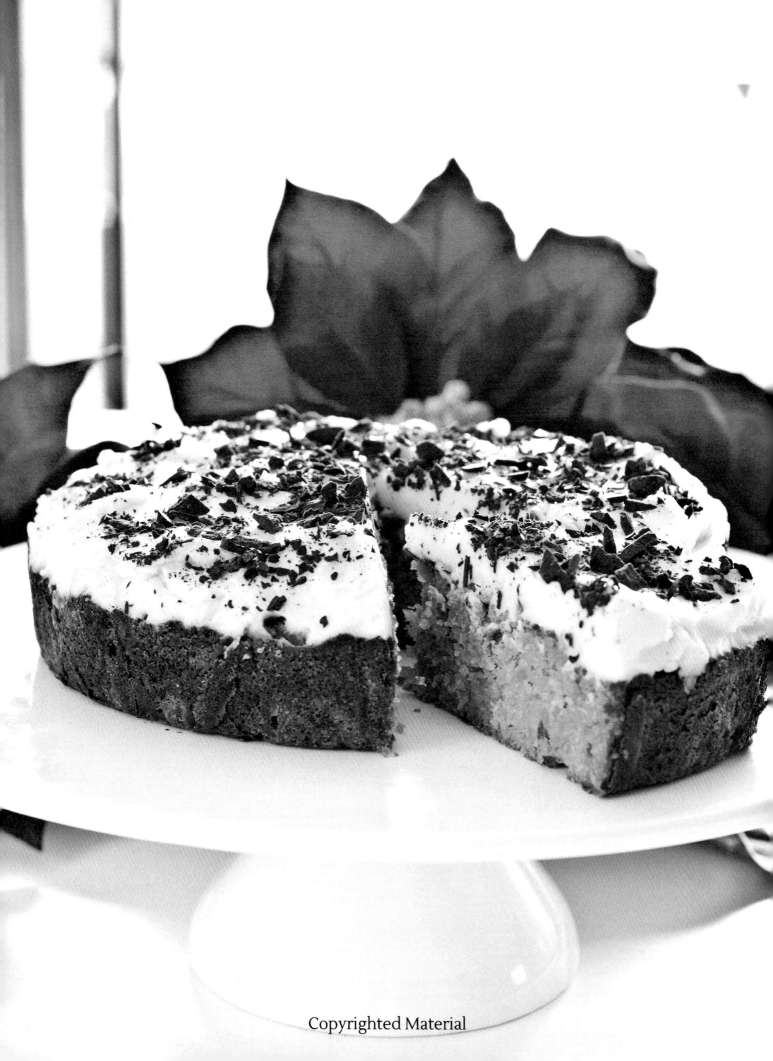

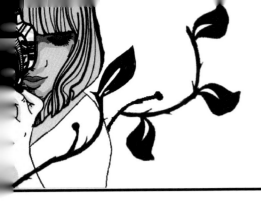

Carrot Cake

For the cake:
1.25 cups oil
1.5 cups sugar
4 eggs
1.3 cups white rice flour
1/3 cup tapioca flour
1/3 cup potato starch
2 tsp cinnamon
1/2 tsp nutmeg
1/2 tsp ginger powder
1.5 tsp baking powder
2 tsp baking soda
1 tsp xantham gum
2.5 cups grated carrots
432gms/15oz can of unsweetened
crushed pineapple, drained
1 cup chopped walnuts

For the icing:
250gms/8.8oz cream cheese
1/2 cup icing sugar
2 tbsp lemon juice

For the cake:
1. Preheat oven to 180°C/350°F.
2. Grease and line a 20cm/8" baking tin.
3. Beat the oil, eggs and sugar until the sugar dissolves.
4. Sift all the dry ingredients together.
5. Add the dry to the wet ingredients and mix well.
6. Add the carrots, walnuts and pineapple and blend in.
7. Pour the mixture into the baking tin.
8. Bake for 55 minutes or until a skewer comes out clean.
9. Leave in the tin for 10 minutes then tip out onto a cooling rack.

For the icing:
10. Blend all the ingredients in a food processor or whip by hand.
11. Smooth the topping over the top of the cake when cold.
12. Sprinkle with grated chocolate if you like.

Note: see page 19 for dairy alternatives

Strands of My Life

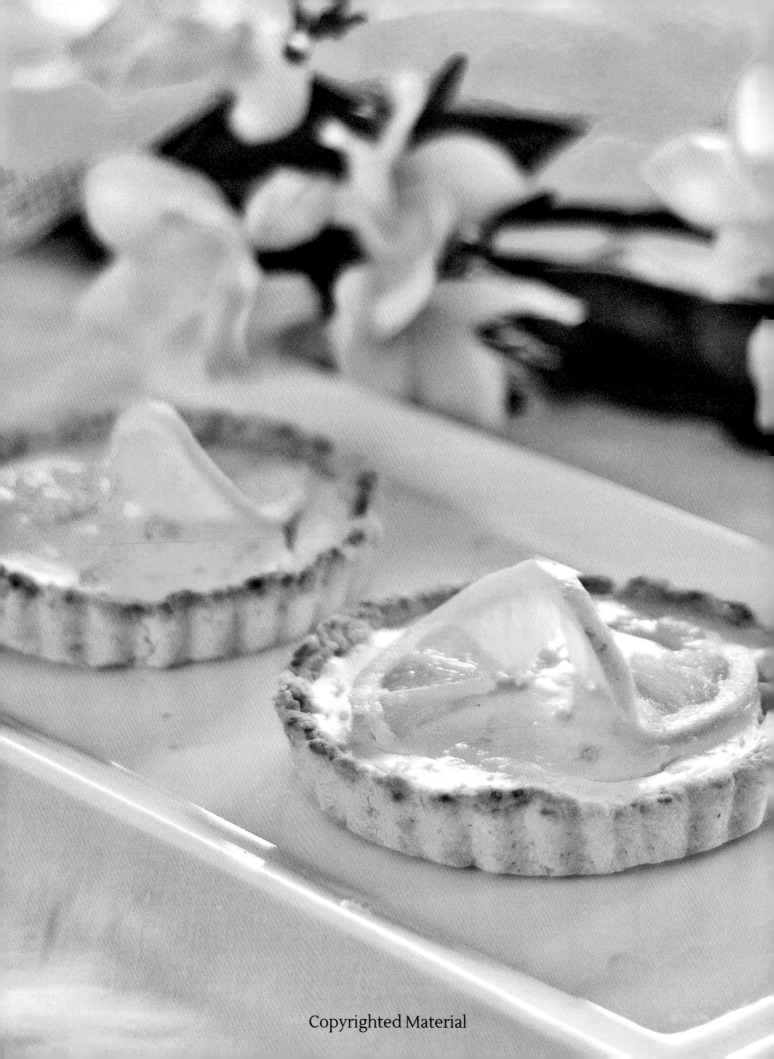

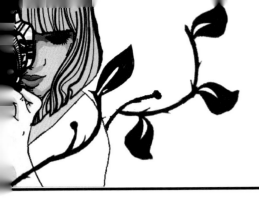

Creamy Lemon Tarts

For the pastry:

3/4 cup white rice flour

1/2 cup potato starch

1/2 cup tapioca flour

1 tbsp sugar

Pinch of salt

120gms/4.2oz butter

1 small egg

2 tsp vinegar

For the filling:

600gms/27oz cream

4 tbsp cane sugar

1/2 cup lemon juice

3 tbsp gelatin

1.5 tbsp tapioca flour

Note: see page 19 for dairy alternatives

For the pastry:
1. Preheat the oven to 350°F/180°C.
2. Mix the flours, salt and sugar in a food processor.
3. Add the cold butter cut up small to the processor and pulse until crumbs form.
4. Whisk egg and vinegar together in a bowl.
5. Add them to the flour/butter mixture and pulse until a dough is formed.
6. If necessary add a little cold water if it is too dry or more white rice flour if it is too wet.
7. Wrap the dough in plastic wrap and place in the fridge for 1 hour.
8. Grease 6 x 11cm/4.25" loose-bottom tart pans.
9. Take a small ball of dough and press out into each tart pan.
10. Prick the base all over with a fork.
11. Place in the oven for about 10 minutes or until browned and cooked through.
12. Remove from the oven and cool in the pans.

For the filling:
13. Bring the cream and sugar to a boil.
14. Add the lemon juice and stir.
15. Dissolve the gelatin in a little hot water and whisk into the mixture.
16. Mix the tapioca flour in a little cold water and add, stirring.
17. Keep stirring until it thickens then take off the heat and let cool.
18. Pour into the cooled pastry shells.
19. Place them in the fridge to set completely.

Strands of My Life

AFTERNOON TEA

Salmon pancake rolls

Smoked chicken mini quiches

Strawberry potato cake

Chocolate zucchini brownies

Lemon marshmallow slice

Coconut & banana cookies

Serves 8

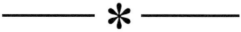

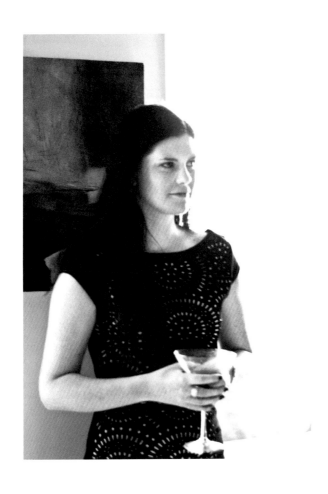
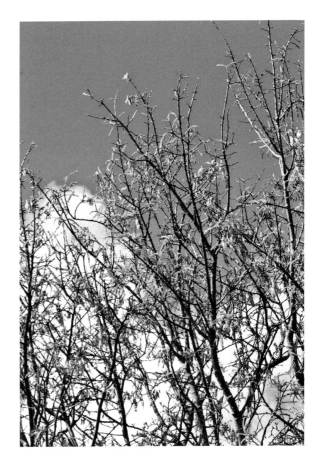
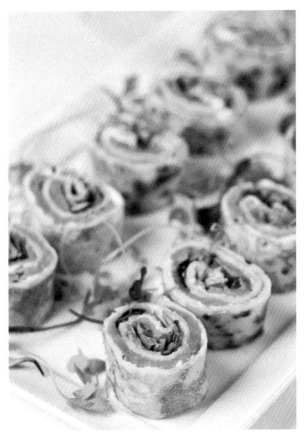
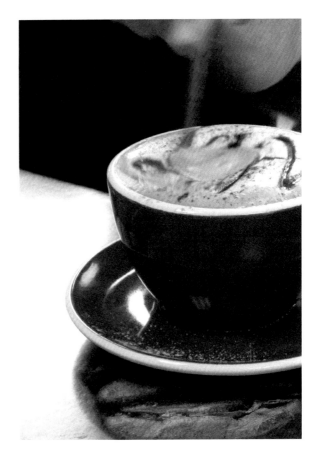

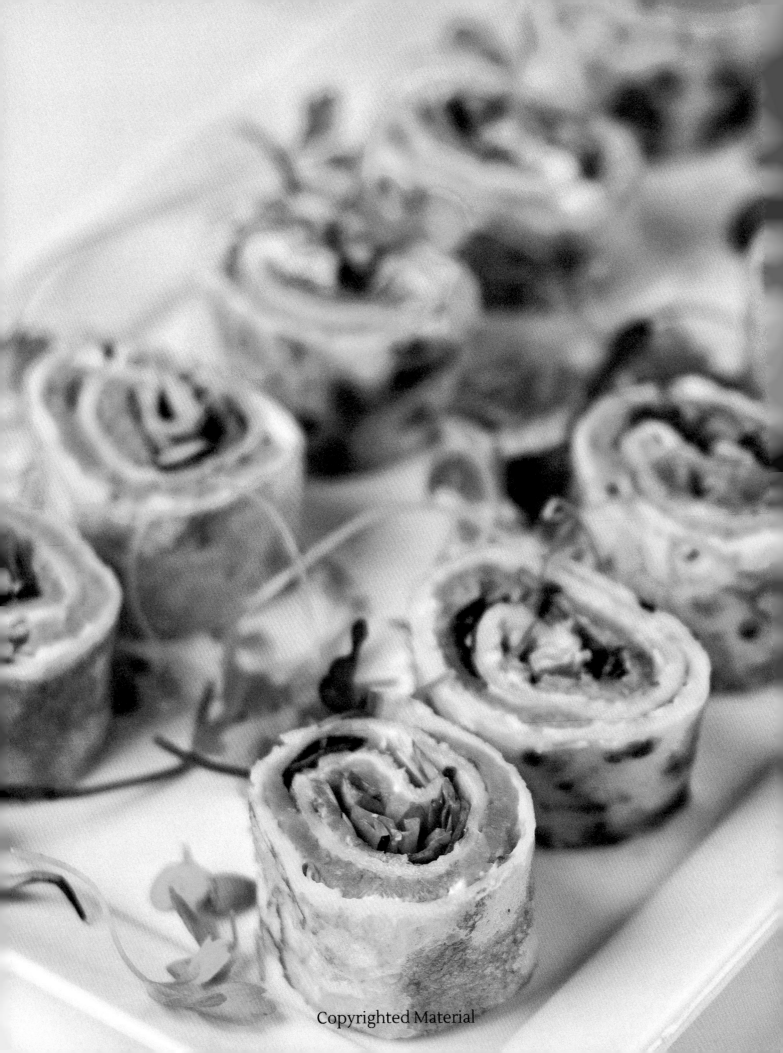

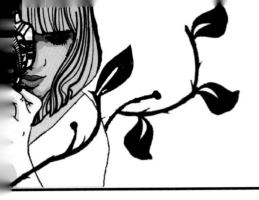

Salmon Pancake Rolls

For the pancakes:

83gms/3oz white rice flour

21gms/.7oz tapioca flour

21gms/.7oz potato starch

Pinch of salt

1 egg

1 cup milk

For the filling:

300gms/10.5oz smoked salmon

100gms/3.5oz cream cheese

Micro herbs or green salad leaves

Note: see page 19 for dairy alternatives

For the pancakes:

1. Sift the flours and salt together.

2. Add the lightly beaten egg and mix as well as possible.

3. Add the milk slowly mixing well in between additions.

4. Melt a little butter in a frying pan and add a thin layer over the base of the pan, moving the pan to cover it evenly.

5. When bubbles form all over the pancake mixture, flip it over and cook on the other side.

6. Repeat with all the mixture. (This should make four quite large ones).

For the filling:

7. Spread the cream cheese over the pancakes, layer the salmon on top and finish with the greens.

8. Roll up the pancakes quite tightly.

9. Slice them into 2.5cm/1" pieces and arrange on a plate.

10. Refrigerate until you need them.

Strands of My Life

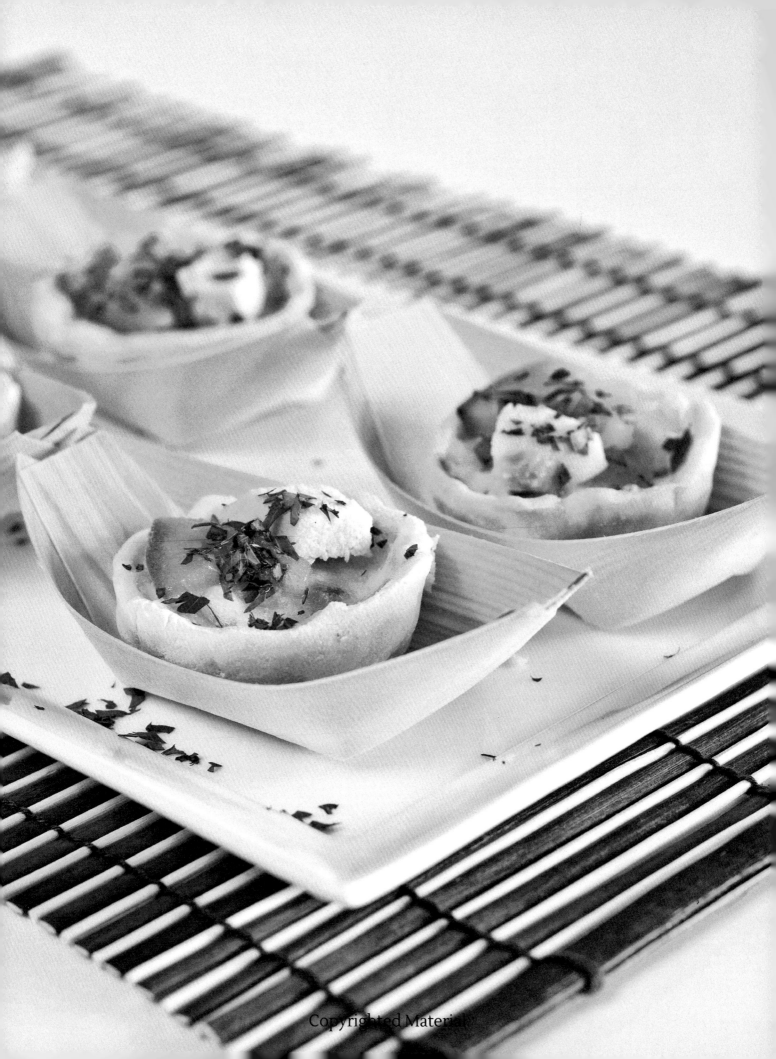

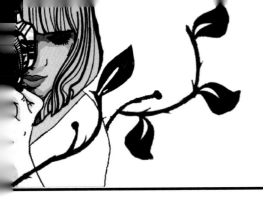

Smoked Chicken Mini Quiches

For the pastry:

1/2 cup white rice flour

3/4 cup brown rice flour

3/4 cup tapioca flour

1/2 tsp baking powder

1/2 tsp salt

30 gms/1 oz butter

3/4 cup water

For the filling:

150 gms/5.3 oz smoked chicken

100 gms/3.5 oz cheese

1 cup cream

3 eggs

salt to taste

Note: see page 19 for dairy alternatives

For the pastry:

1. Mix all the dry ingredients together in a bowl.

2. Rub the butter into the dry ingredients until a crumbly mixture is formed.

3. Add the water and mix to form a dough.

4. Place in the fridge for 30 minutes.

5. Heat oven to 180°C/350°F.

6. Oil a 20-capacity muffin tin.

7. Roll out the chilled dough on a floured surface and cut out circles the size of your muffin tins.

8. Press into the muffin tin moulds and trim edges.

9. Bake for 10 minutes then remove.

For the filling:

10. Chop up the smoked chicken into small pieces and place in the pastry cases.

11. Grate the cheese and place on top of the chicken.

12. Beat together the eggs, cream and salt.

13. Pour over the cheese until the cases are full.

14. Place in the oven for about 10 minutes until set.

15. Decorate with pieces of tomato and chicken and sprinkle with chopped parsley.

Strands of My Life

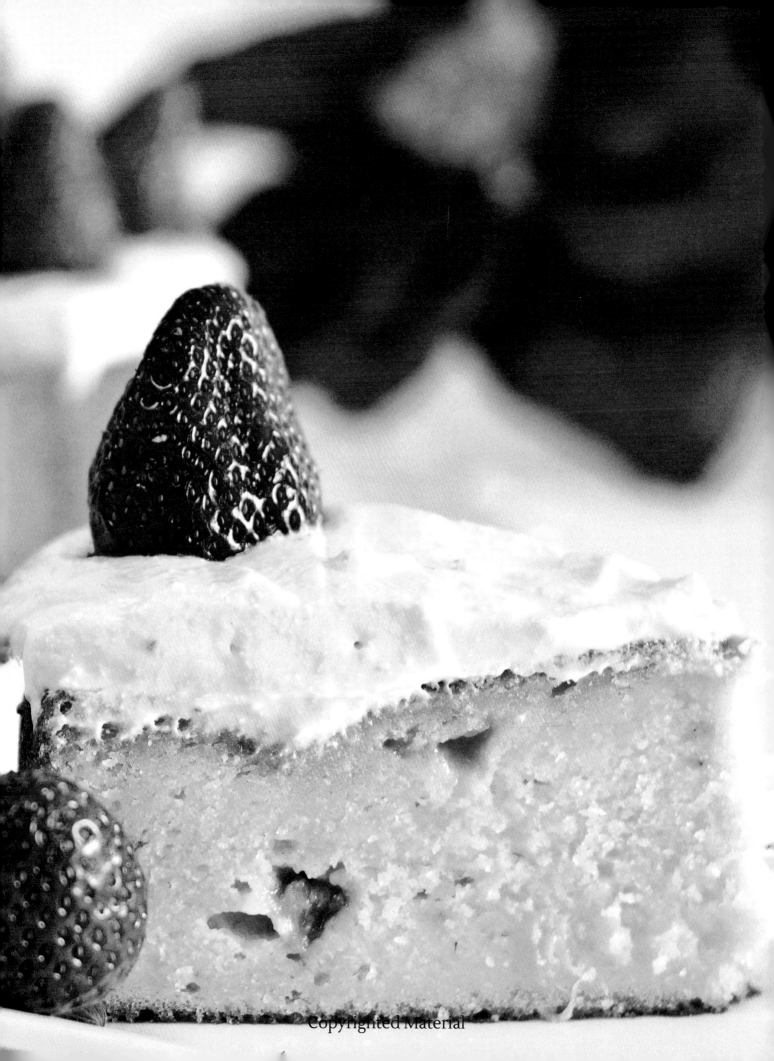

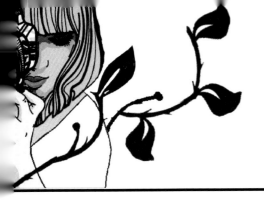

Strawberry Potato Cake

For the cake:

200gms/7oz softened butter

150gms/5.5oz caster sugar

4 eggs

110gms/3.9oz white rice flour

29gms/1oz potato starch

30gms/1oz tapioca flour

250gms/8.8oz mashed potato

10 strawberries

2 tsp baking powder

For the syrup:

1 tbsp caster sugar

8 big strawberries

1 tbsp water

For the topping:

200gms/7oz cream cheese

200gms/7oz cottage cheese

1 tbsp icing sugar

2 tbsp strawberry syrup

For the cake:

1. Preheat the oven to 180°C/350°F.

2. Butter and line a 20cm/8" cake tin.

3. Beat the sugar and butter together until light and fluffy.

4. Add the eggs one at a time while still beating.

5. Sift the flours and baking powder together and add to the wet ingredients.

6. Add the mashed potato and chopped strawberries and mix through.

7. Pour into the tin and bake for 35-40 minutes or until a skewer comes out clean.

8. Cool a little then tip out onto a wire rack.

9. Pour the syrup slowly over the warm cake and rub into the top.

10. Cool completely before piling the topping on.

For the syrup:

11. Place all ingredients into a food processor and blend until a thin puree is formed. Reserve 2 tbsp for the topping.

For the topping:

12. Place all ingredients into a food processor and blend until a thick cream is formed.

Note: see page 19 for dairy alternatives

Strands of My Life

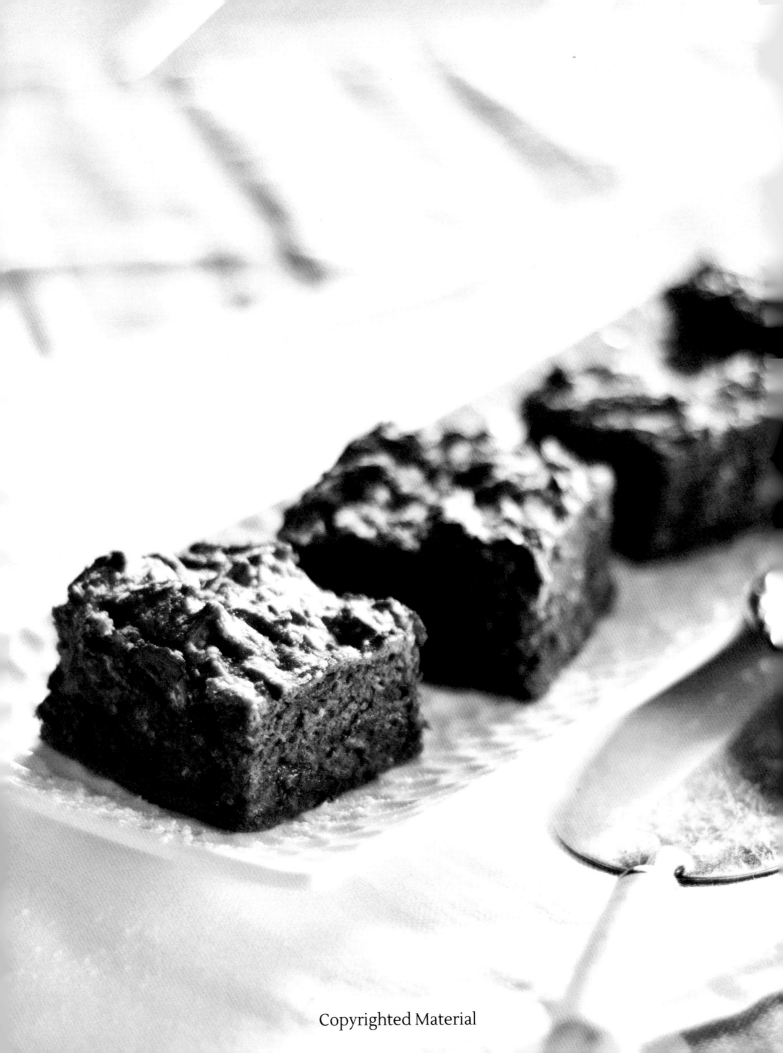

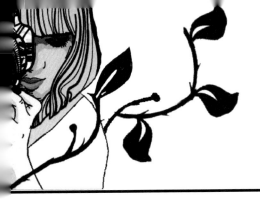

Chocolate
Zucchini Brownies

1¼ cup white rice flour

¼ cup tapioca flour

¼ cup potato starch

1/2 tsp salt

1.5 tsp baking powder

1/2 tsp cinnamon

1/2 cup cocoa powder

2 eggs

115g/4oz butter, softened

1.3 cup cane sugar

1 tsp vanilla

2 cups grated zucchini

1 cup chopped dark chocolate

1. Preheat the oven to 350°F or 180°C.

2. Mix all the dry ingredients except the sugar in a large bowl.

3. Place the butter, vanilla essence, sugar and eggs in a food processor and process to bind.

4. Grate the zucchini and squeeze to remove as much of the liquid as possible.

5. Add the zucchini and chocolate to the wet mixture.

6. Add the wet mixture to the dry and blend well.

7. Spoon the batter into a 17.5 x 27.5cm or 7 inch x 11 inch baking tin.

8. Bake for 20-30 minutes or until a toothpick comes out clean.

9. Cool, tip out of the tin onto a board and cut into squares.

(Note: eat only one at a sitting.)

Strands of My Life

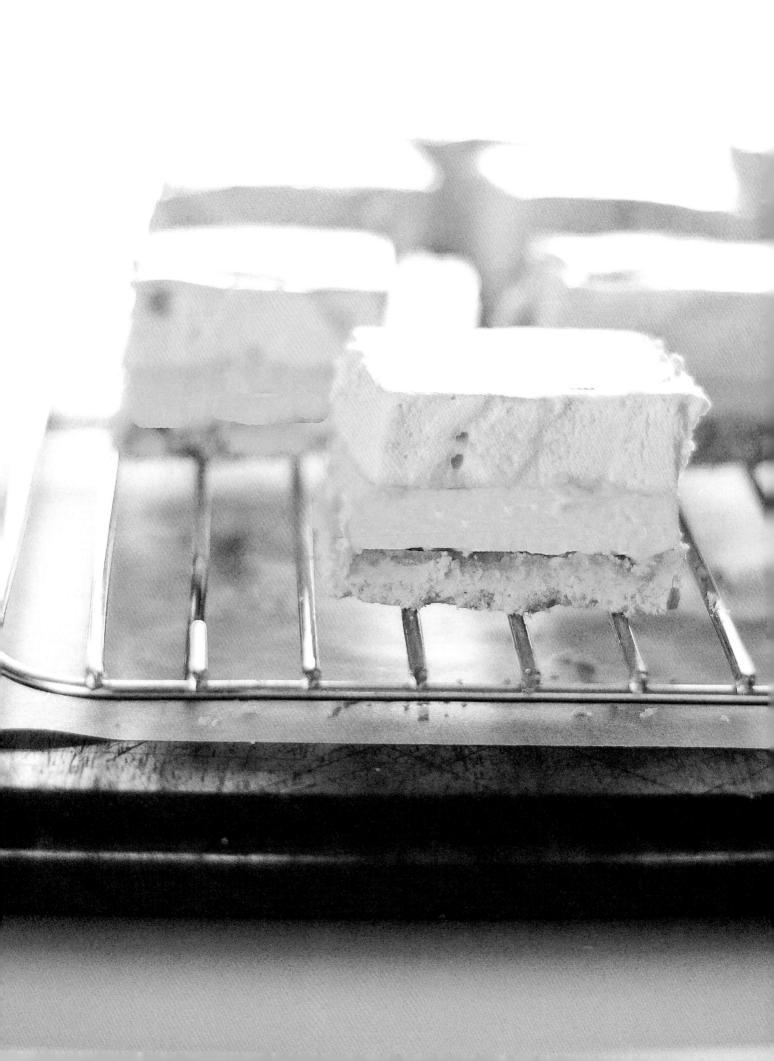

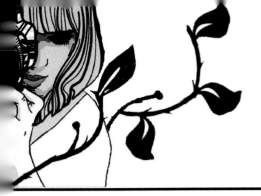

Lemon Marshmallow Slice

For the base:

½ cup of white rice flour

¼ cup tapioca flour

¼ cup potato starch

2 tsp cane sugar

pinch of salt

80gms/2.75oz chilled butter

1 egg

2 tsp cider vinegar

For the lemon layer:

400mls/13.5oz cream

3 tbsp cane sugar

1/3 cup lemon juice

2 tbsp gelatin

1 tbsp tapioca flour

For the marshmallow:

2 tbsp gelatin

1/4 cup water

1.5 cups cane sugar

1 cup water

1 tsp vanilla

Note: see page 19 for dairy alternatives

For the base:

1. Preheat the oven to 180°C/350°F.
2. In a food processor, add the flours, sugar, salt and butter, cut up small. Process until crumbs form.
3. Whisk together the egg and vinegar.
4. Add to the processor and process again until a firm dough forms. Adjust with a little cold water or a little more flour if necessary.
5. Butter and line a 17.5 x 27.5cm/7" x 11" slice tin.
6. Press the dough into the prepared tin.
7. Place in the oven for 10 minutes or until golden.
8. Cool completely.

For the lemon layer:

1. Bring the cream and sugar to the boil.
2. Add the lemon juice and stir.
3. Dissolve the gelatine 1 tbsp hot water and add. Whisk.
4. Mix the tapioca flour in a little cold water and add.
5. Keep stirring until it thickens then take off the heat and let cool.
6. Pour it over the cooled base and place in the fridge to set completely.

For the marshmallow:

1. Place everything in a saucepan and bring to the boil, stirring.
2. Let boil, not stirring, for 15 minutes, then cool to lukewarm.
3. With egg beaters, whisk until thick.
4. Pour onto the set lemon layer and place in the fridge to firm up.
5. Once set completely, cut into slices.

Strands of My Life

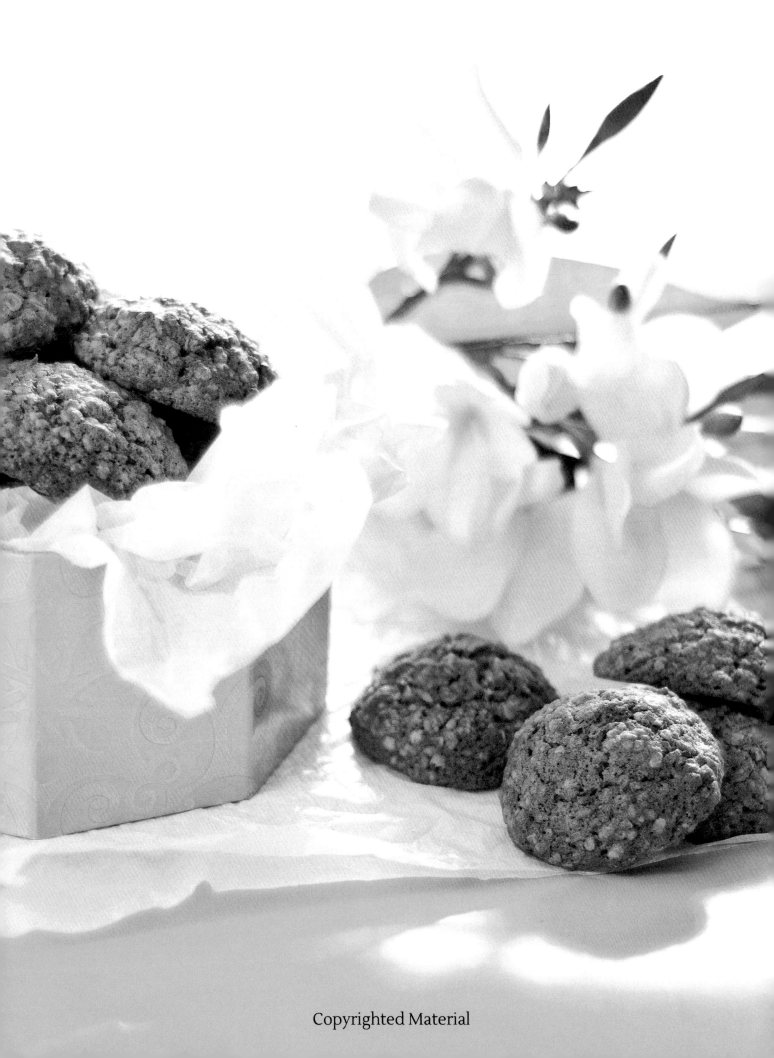

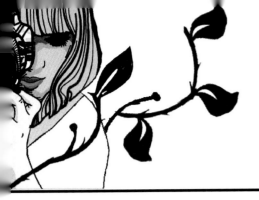

Coconut Banana Cookies

1/4 cup coconut flour

1/2 cup oil

2 tbsp sugar

1 ripe banana

2 eggs

1 tsp cinnamon

1 tsp vanilla

pinch salt

1/2 tsp baking soda

1 cup coconut

1. Heat the oven to 350°F/180°C.
2. Mix the dry ingredients, oil, banana and sugar in a food processor.
3. Add the eggs and vanilla and mix.
4. Remove the mixture from the food processor to a bowl and add the coconut.
5. Place a sheet of baking paper on an oven tray.
6. Drop big spoonfuls of the dough onto the paper and shape them into circles.
7. Bake about 10 minutes until they are golden but still soft.
8. Remove from the oven and leave to cool on the tray for half an hour so they firm up a little.

Note: 1/4 cup shredded coconut is low Fodmap

Strands of My Life

DINNER WITH FRIENDS

Courgette fritters

Lamb kofta & potato rosti

Chia seed bread

Strawberry sour cream tart

Serves 6

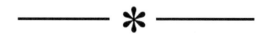

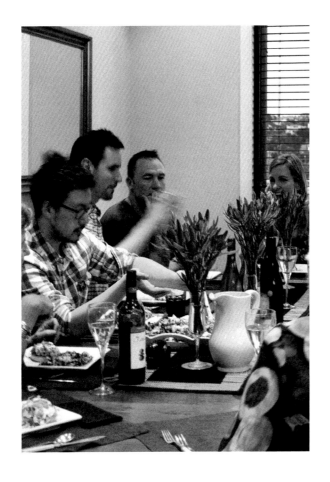

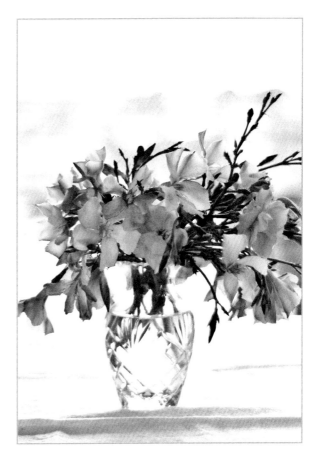

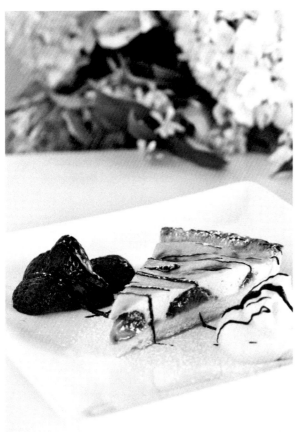

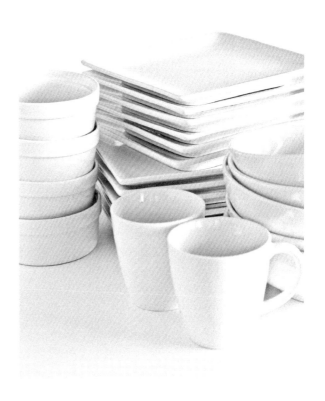

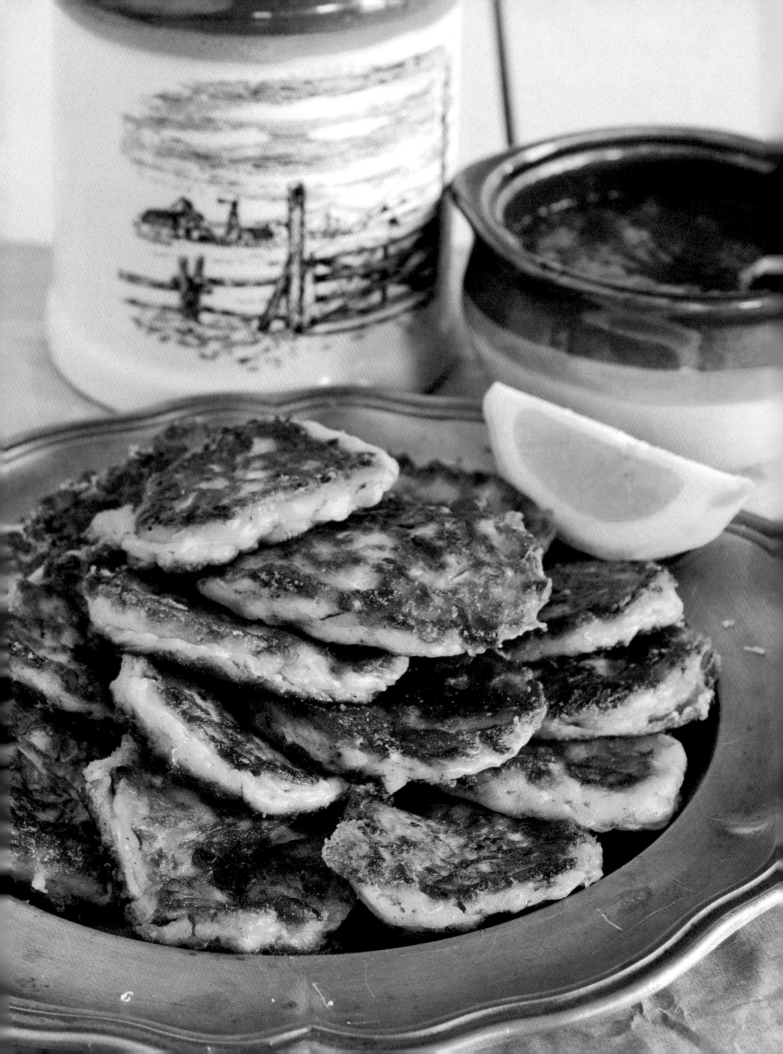

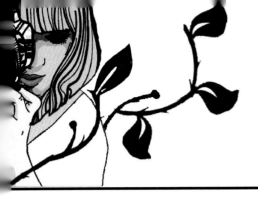

Zucchini Fritters

¾ cup white rice flour

¼ cup tapioca flour

2 tsp baking powder

½ tsp salt

½ tsp black pepper

2 eggs

1 cup milk

1 cup grated zucchini

1 cup grated cheese

¼ cup chopped chives

Note: see page 19 for dairy alternatives

1. Combine flours, baking powder, salt and pepper in a bowl.

2. Beat the eggs and milk together.

3. Stir into the flour mixture to make a batter.

4. Squeeze excess juice out of the grated zucchini.

5. Stir the zucchini, cheese and chives into the batter.

6. Heat a little oil in a frying pan.

7. Cook spoonfuls of the mixture over a medium heat until golden on one side.

8. Turn and cook the other side.

9. Place the fritters on a platter and keep warm while cooking the remaining batter.

10. Serve with chilli sauce (no garlic),

Strands of My Life

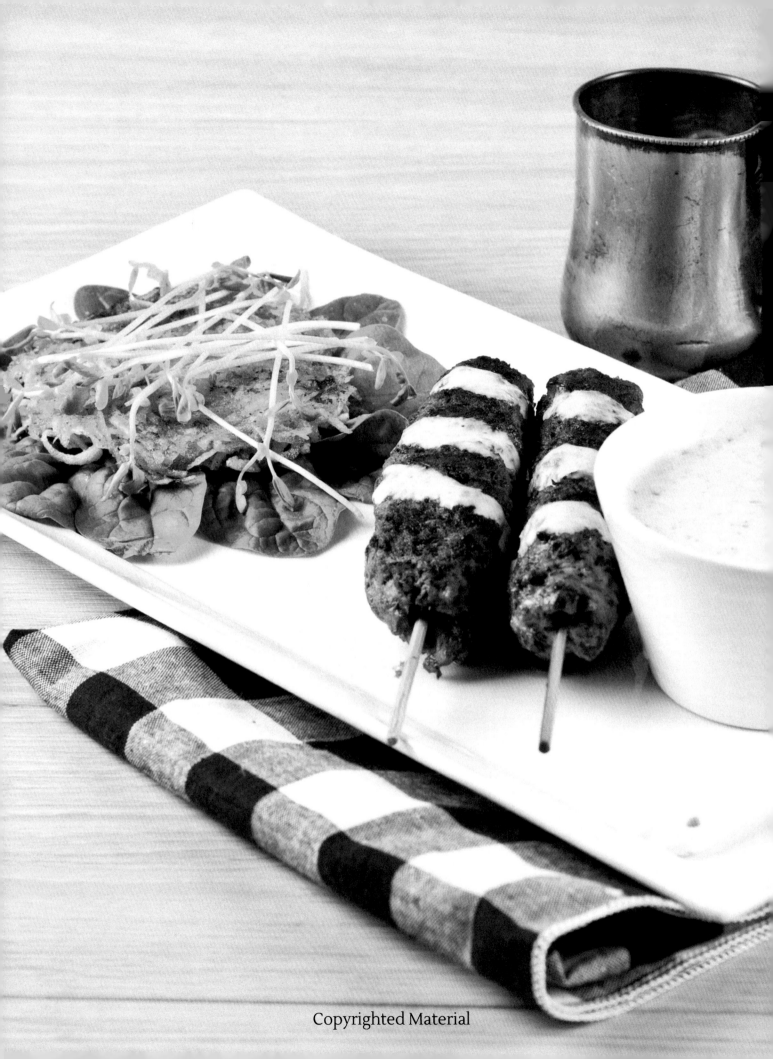

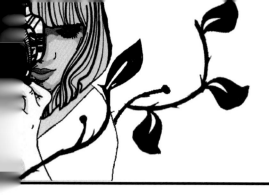

Lamb Kofta & Potato Rosti

For the lamb kofta:

750gms/26.5 oz minced lamb

Small bunch of parsley, chopped

2 red chilli, minced

2 tsp turmeric

2 tsp coriander powder

2 tsp cumin seeds

Salt & pepper

For the potato rosti:

4 large potatoes

Salt & pepper

For the sauce:

8 tbsp plain yoghurt

Small bunch of mint, chopped

1 tsp cumin powder

Squeeze of lemon juice

Salt & pepper

Note: see page 19 for dairy alternatives

For the lamb kofta:

1. Mix all the ingredients together.

2. Shape into 6 long sausages and insert wooden skewers into them.

3. Place on a heated, oiled grill and cook until done, turning a few times.

For the potato rosti:

4. Peel the potatoes, then pass them through the grate function of a food processor.

5. Squeeze all the liquid out of the grated potato.

6. Season with salt and pepper.

7. Heat a mixture of oil and butter in a frying pan.

8. Place big spoonfuls of the potato in the pan and flatten as well as shape them into rounds.

9. Cook well until browned, then turn and cook on the other side. Don't have the heat too high or they will brown before they are cooked through.

10. Remove from the pan and place on paper towels to absorb some of the oil.

For the sauce:

11. Combine all of the ingredients and place in a small bowl to serve with the lamb.

Strands of My Life

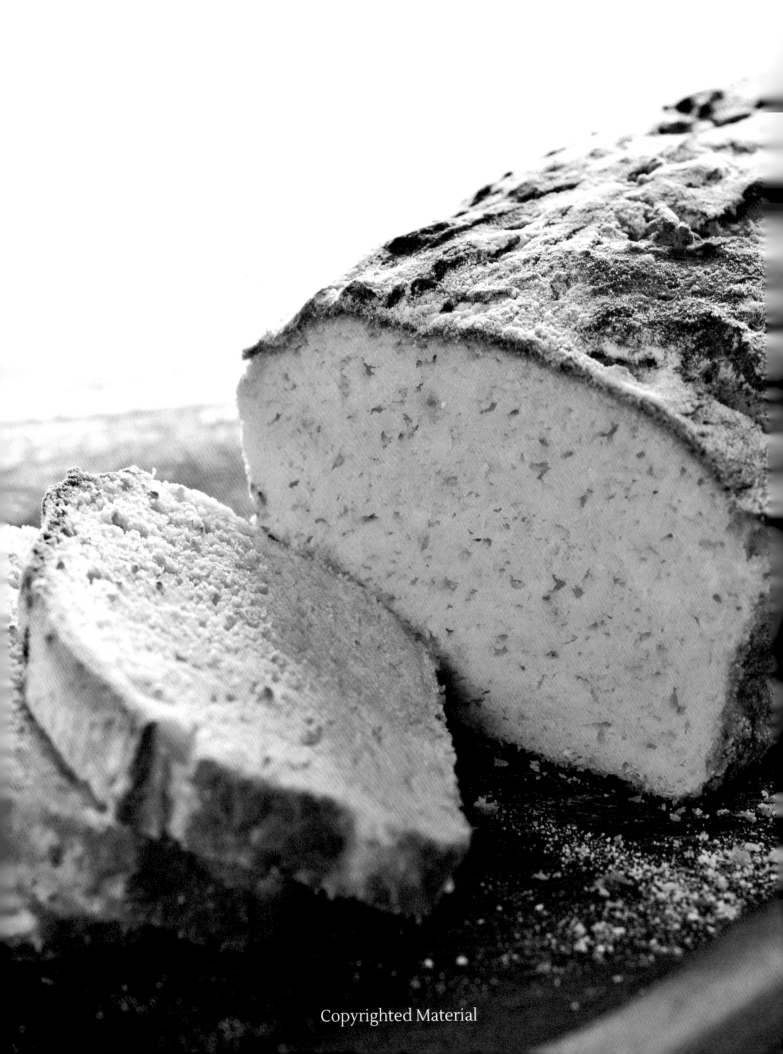

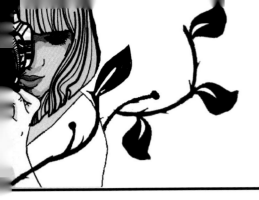

Chia Seed Bread

1.5 cups white rice flour

1/2 cup brown rice flour

1/2 cup potato starch

3/4 cup tapioca flour

2 tbsp chia seeds

1 tsp salt

3 eggs

3 tbsp olive oil

1 cup warm water

1 tbsp sugar

1 tsp white wine vinegar

2 tsp fresh yeast granules

1. Place everything in a breadmaker and put it on the dough setting. or blend everything by hand.

2. When it is mixed, place it in an oiled loaf tin in the drawer under the oven for 1 hour.

3. Halfway through the rising, preheat the oven to 180°C/350°F. This will help the dough below to rise.

4. Bake the loaf for 30 minutes or until it sounds hollow when you knock the top with a knuckle.

5. Let sit in the loaf tin for 5 mins and then remove to a cooling rack.

6. Let cool completely before slicing.

Strands of My Life

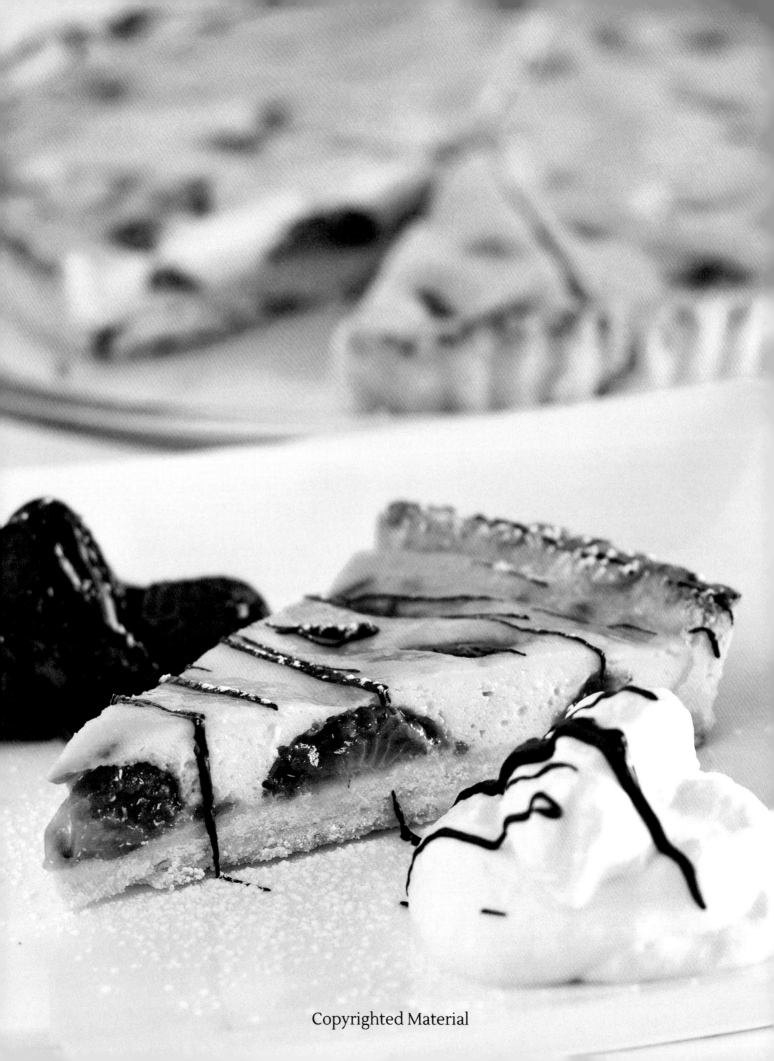

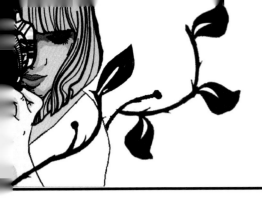

Strawberry Sour Cream Tart

For the pastry:

133gms/4.7oz white rice flour

22gms/0.8oz tapioca flour

45gms/1.6oz potato starch

pinch of salt

1 heaped tbsp sugar

100gms/3.5oz butter

1 medium egg

For the filling:

200gms/7oz fresh strawberries

2 tsp tapioca flour

300gms/10.5 oz sour cream

1/2 cup icing sugar

3 egg yolks

2 tbsp white rice flour

Note: see page 19 for dairy alternatives

For the pastry:

1. Blend all the dry ingredients in a food processor.

2. Add the butter cut into small pieces to the food processor and process until fine crumbs form.

3. Add the egg and process until it forms a dough.

4. Remove from the processor and add a little more rice flour if it is too wet – this depends on the size of your egg.

5. Press into a greased tart dish and place in the fridge for 30 mins.

6. Preheat the oven to 180°C/360°F.

7. Place baking paper in the base of the tart crust and fill with rice or dried beans and blind bake for 15 minutes.

8. Remove the paper and beans/rice and cook for another 10 mins.

For the filling:

9. Mix the strawberries in the tapioca flour and place in the pastry case.

10. Combine remaining ingredients together and whisk until smooth.

11. Pour over the strawberries.

12. Bake at 160°C/320°F for 45 mins or until set.

13. Allow to cool for 10 mins before removing from the tin.

14. Drizzle with chocolate if you like, and dust with icing sugar and serve.

Strands of My Life

FORMAL DINNER PARTY

Prawn & courgette appetizers

Lamb rack

Roasted vegetables

Chocolate mousse meringue desserts

Serves 6

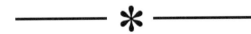

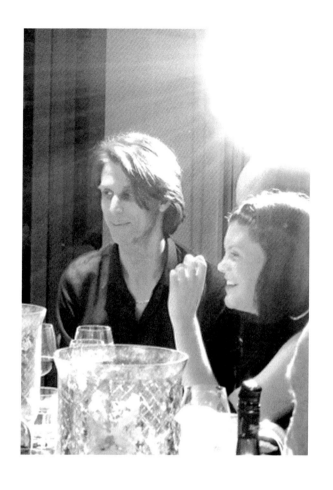 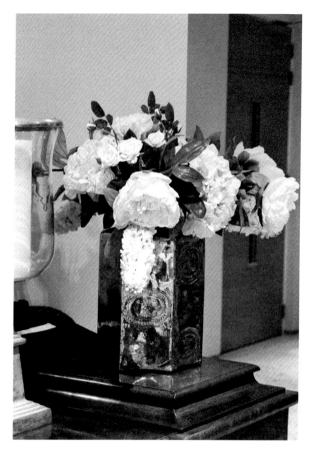

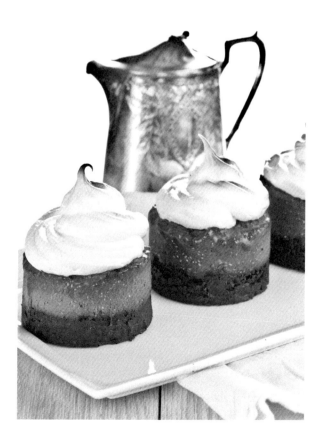 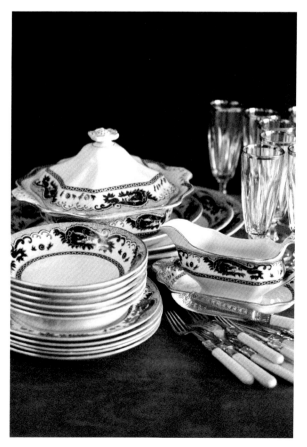

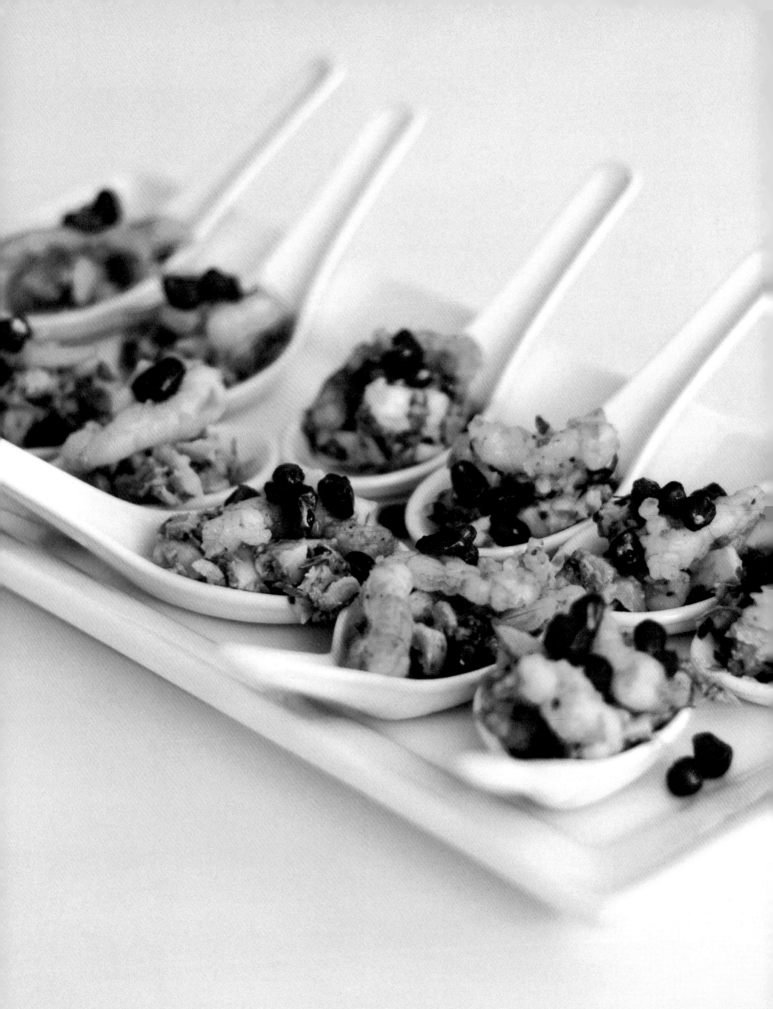

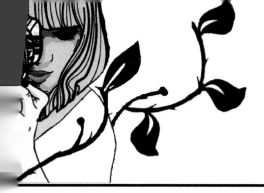

Prawn & Zucchini Spoonfuls

3 zucchini

1 tbsp cream cheese

2 tbsp parsley

1 tsp garlic-infused olive oil

Salt & pepper

2 uncooked, peeled prawns per spoon

1 tbsp butter

1 tsp garlic-infused olive oil

Lemon juice

Pomegranate Seeds

Note: see page 19 for dairy alternatives

1. Chop up the zucchini finely and fry in a little rice bran oil and the garlic-infused olive oil until soft.

2. Add the cream cheese and season.

3. Finely chop the parsley and add to the zucchini.

4. Quickly fry the prawns in the butter and garlic oil until just cooked.

5. Squeeze a little lemon juice over them.

6. Almost fill the spoons with the courgette mixture.

7. Place 2 prawns on top.

8. Sprinkle over the pomegranate seeds and serve warm.

Strands of My Life

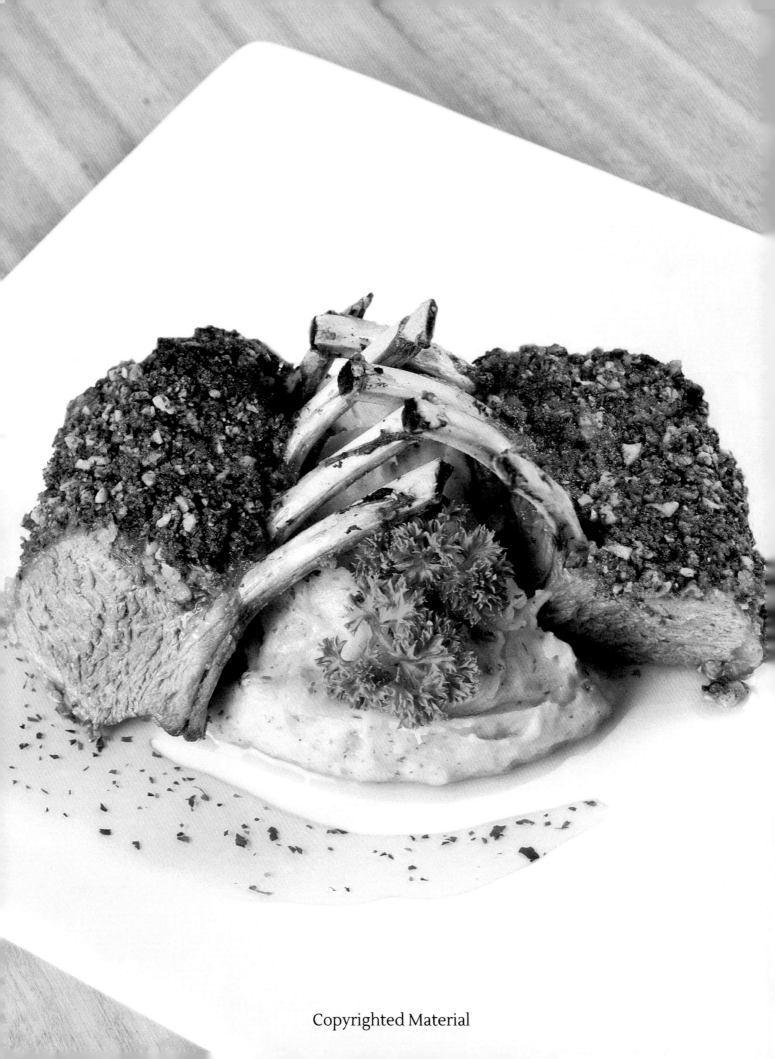

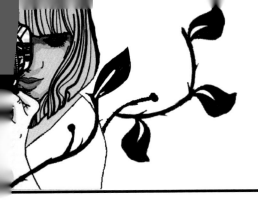

Crusted Rack of Lamb

3 medium or 6 small racks of lamb

2 tbsp dijon mustard

1 cup of packed parsley

1 tsp smoked paprika

Zest of 1 lemon

1/4 cup slivered walnuts

1 cup fresh gluten-free breadcrumbs

2-3 tbsp garlic-infused olive oil

Salt & pepper

1. Preheat the oven to 180°C/350°F.

2. Season the meat.

3. Heat a frying pan with a little olive oil and brown the racks on both sides. Cool a little.

4. For the crust, put the parsley, paprika and zest in a food processor and chop finely.

5. Add the walnuts, breadcrumbs and oil and pulse to combine.

6. Spread the top of the racks with the mustard and press on the breadcrumb mixture.

7. Roast for 20-25 minutes for medium rare lamb.

8. Rest loosely covered for 5 minutes before carving.

9. Serve with mint sauce, simple pureed potatoes with a little parsley and the roasted vegetables in the next recipe.

Strands of My Life

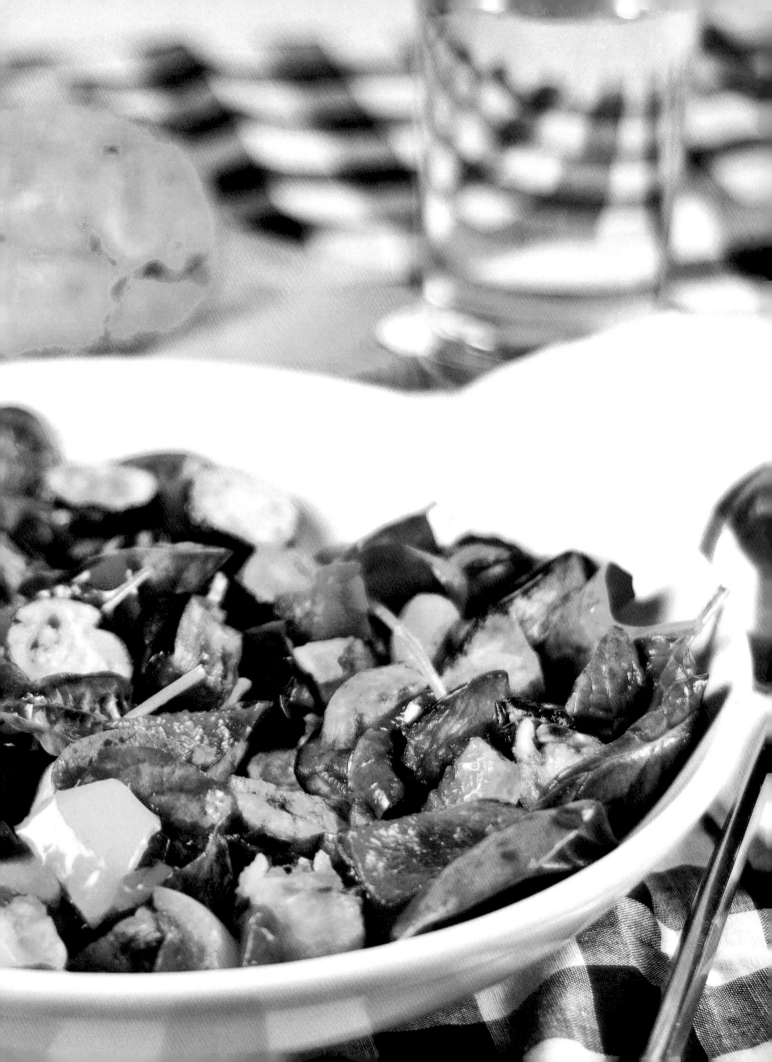

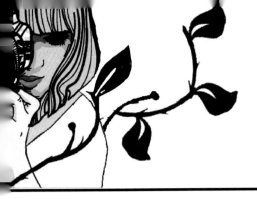

Roasted Vegetables

For the vegetables:

1 eggplant, cut up

2 zucchini, sliced

1 red capsicum, cut up

1 yellow capsicum, cut up

1/2 a pumpkin, cut up small

Garlic-infused olive oil

Salt and pepper

A bunch of baby spinach

2 spring onions (green part only)

Small bunch of parsley, chopped

1 red chilli, chopped

For the salad:

1. Preheat the oven to 350°F or 180°C.

2. Place all the cut up vegetables (except the spinach) in a large bowl.

3. Drizzle with the oil, season well and mix.

4. Spread the vegetables out over two baking trays and place in the heated oven for 20 minutes until golden and cooked.

5. Remove from the oven and add the spinach leaves, parsley, chilli and chopped up spring onions. Toss together.

6. Serve hot.

Note: 1/4 cup of eggplant is low Fodmap

Strands of My Life

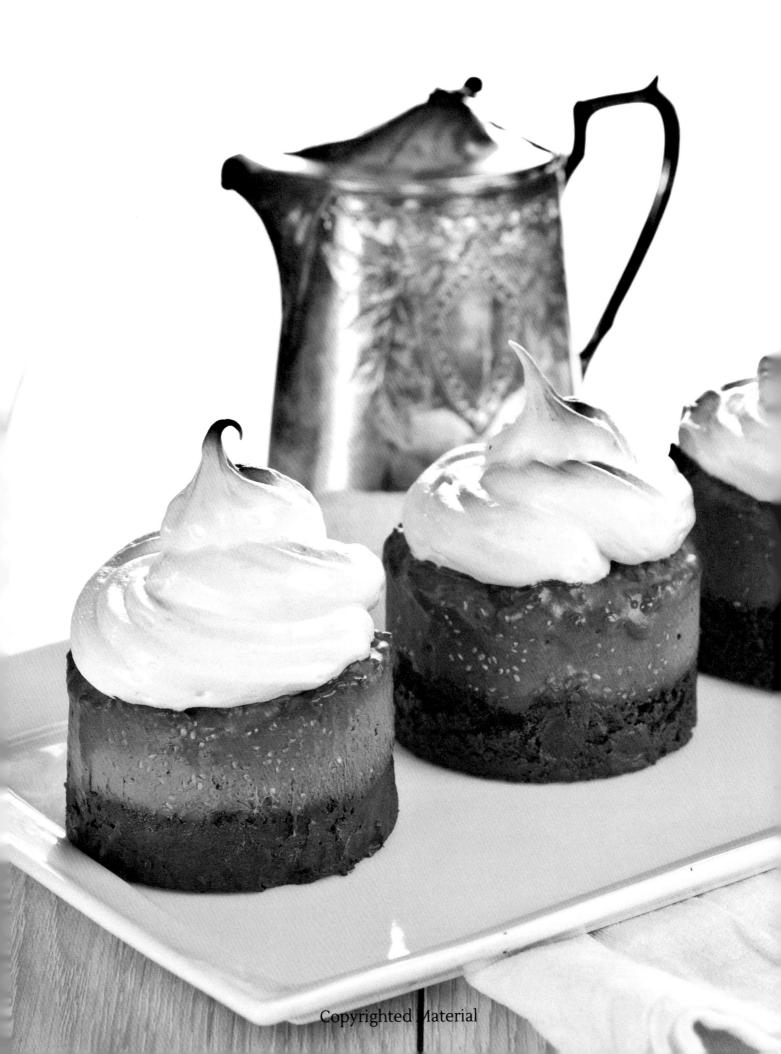

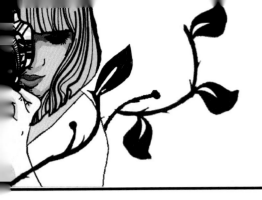

Chocolate Mousse Meringue Desserts

For the base:

Use the brownie recipe on page 63.

For the mousse:

1 cup cocoa

6 tbsp cane sugar

2.25 cups coconut milk

6 tbsp chia seeds

For the meringue:

3 large egg whites

165gms/5.8oz caster sugar

For the mousse:

1. Place everything in a food processor and process until smooth.

For the meringue:

2. Whisk the egg whites until soft peaks are formed.

3. Gradually add the sugar while beating and continue beating until stiff peaks form and the egg whites are thick and glossy.

To assemble the cake:

4. Cut rounds out of the brownie base with your 7.5cm/3" moulds.

5. Place the moulds with the base inside in a lined baking dish with plenty of space.

6. Fill to the top with the mousse and place in the fridge to set well.

7. Once the mousse is set, run a warm knife around the inside of the mould and slide the mould off leaving the cakes in the baking dish.

8. Make the meringue and pipe on top of the cakes.

9. Place under a warm grill for a short time until toasted. Don't take your eyes off them or they will burn.

10. Place in the fridge immediately to firm up again.

(Note: Make these small or eat only half a one of these.)

Strands of My Life

FAMILY DINNER

Hamburgers

Panzanella salad

Lemon tart

Serves 6

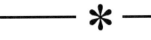

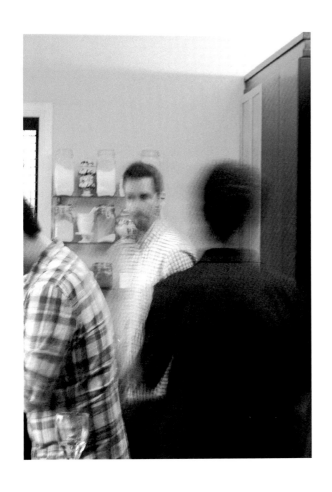

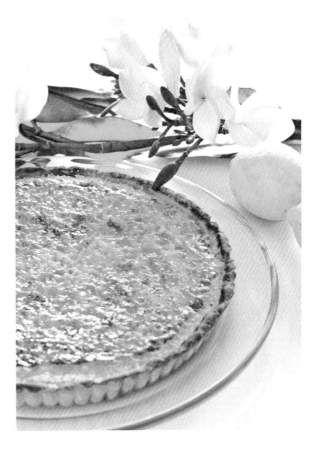

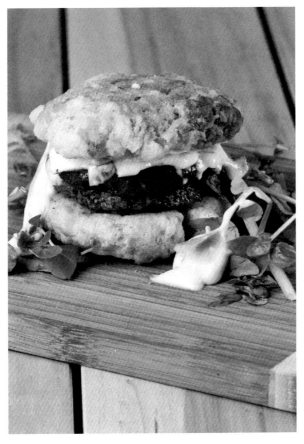

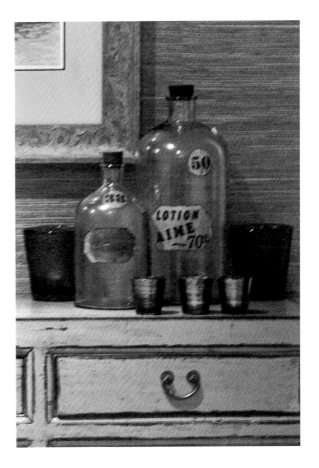

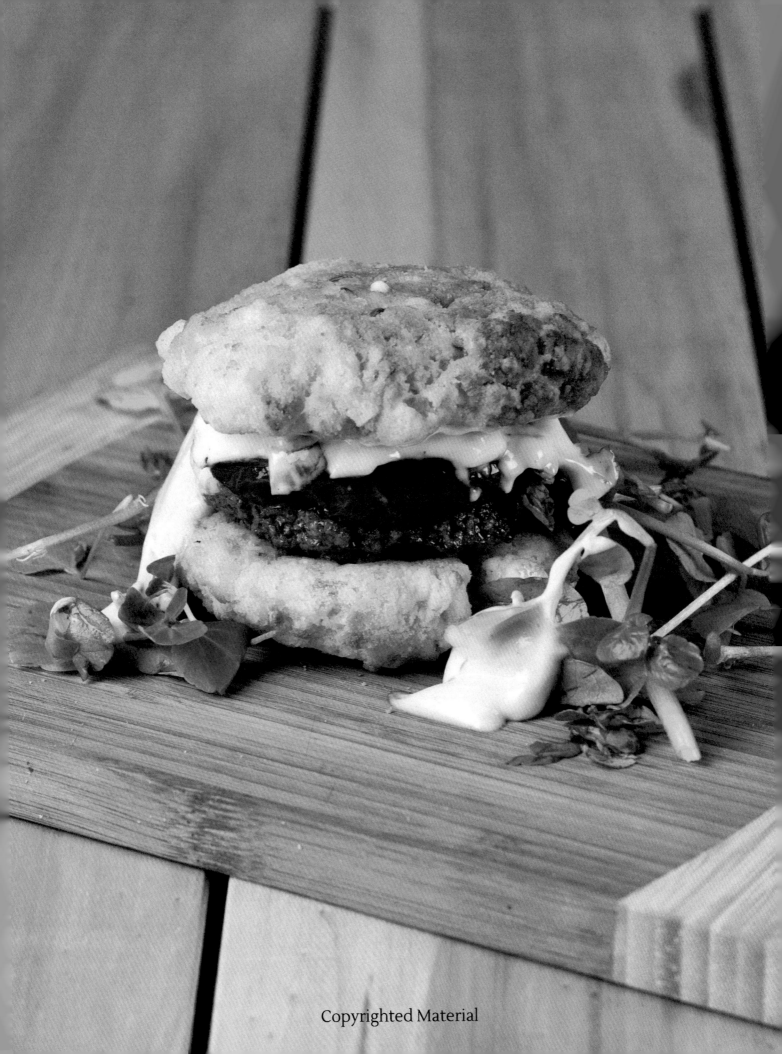

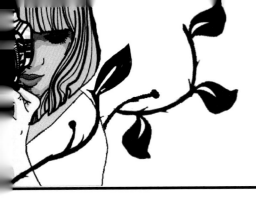

Hamburgers

For the buns:
2/3 cup of olive oil
1 cup of water
1 tsp salt
1.5 cup of tapioca flour
1.5 cup of white rice flour
2 eggs
2 tsp of cumin seeds

For the burgers:
750gms/26.5oz minced meat
Salt & pepper
2 tsp cumin powder

For the mayonnaise:
1 egg
2 tbsp lemon juice
½ tsp salt
½ tsp black pepper
½ tsp dried mustard
¼ pt/118ml rice bran oil
¼ pt/118ml olive oil

To assemble:
Water cress
Roasted or fresh tomatoes

For the buns:

1. Sift the two flours and salt together. Add the cumin seeds.

2. In a bowl, whisk the olive oil, eggs and water well.

3. Mix the wet and dry ingredients together and knead to form a dough.

4. Divide into 6 pieces and mound them into a burger bun shape. (They won't change size.)

5. Place the rolls on baking paper on an oven tray and bake at 350°/180°C for 35 - 40 minutes.

For the burgers:

6. Mix the ingredients together and shape into 6 burgers.

7. Oil a grill lightly and grill the burgers on both sides until cooked.

For the mayonnaise:

8. Put everything except the oil into a food processor and blend for a few seconds.

9. Keep the machine going and slowly add the mixed oils in a thin stream until the mixture thickens.

To assemble:

10. Split the buns open and spread a thin layer of mayonnaise over them.

11. Place the freshly cooked burger on one side and top with the tomato and watercress.

12. Drizzle with more mayonnaise and top with the other half of the bun.

Strands of My Life

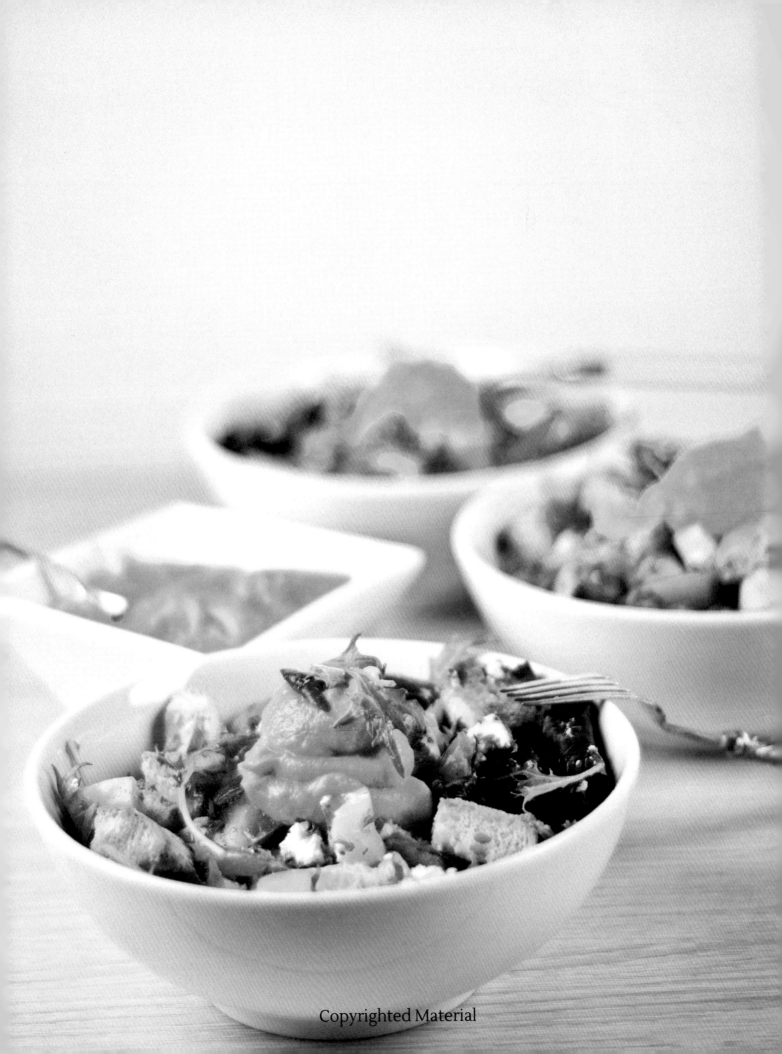

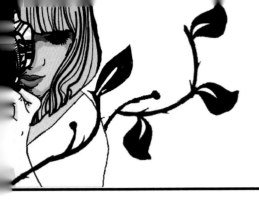

Panzanella Salad

2 tomatoes - cut up

3 spring onions (green part only) - sliced

Yellow pepper – diced

1 stick of celery – sliced up small

Parsley, chopped – not too finely

A handful of green salad leaves

100g/3.5oz feta cheese – crumbled

6 slices of gluten-free bread (See pg 75)

1 red chilli – chopped up small

1 cup pumpkin puree

1 cup coconut milk

1 tsp dijon mustard

Juice of 1 lemon

1 tsp garlic-infused olive oil

Salt & pepper to taste

1. Turn the oven on to 350°F/180°C.
2. Cube the bread and place on an oven tray and bake for 15 minutes. You could drizzle them with olive oil but the dressing will do the job.
3. Chop and dice the vegetables as instructed in the ingredients.
4. Place in a large bowl together with the feta.
5. Add the croutons.
6. Mix the last 6 ingredients with a whisk and serve with the salad as a thick dressing.

Strands of My Life

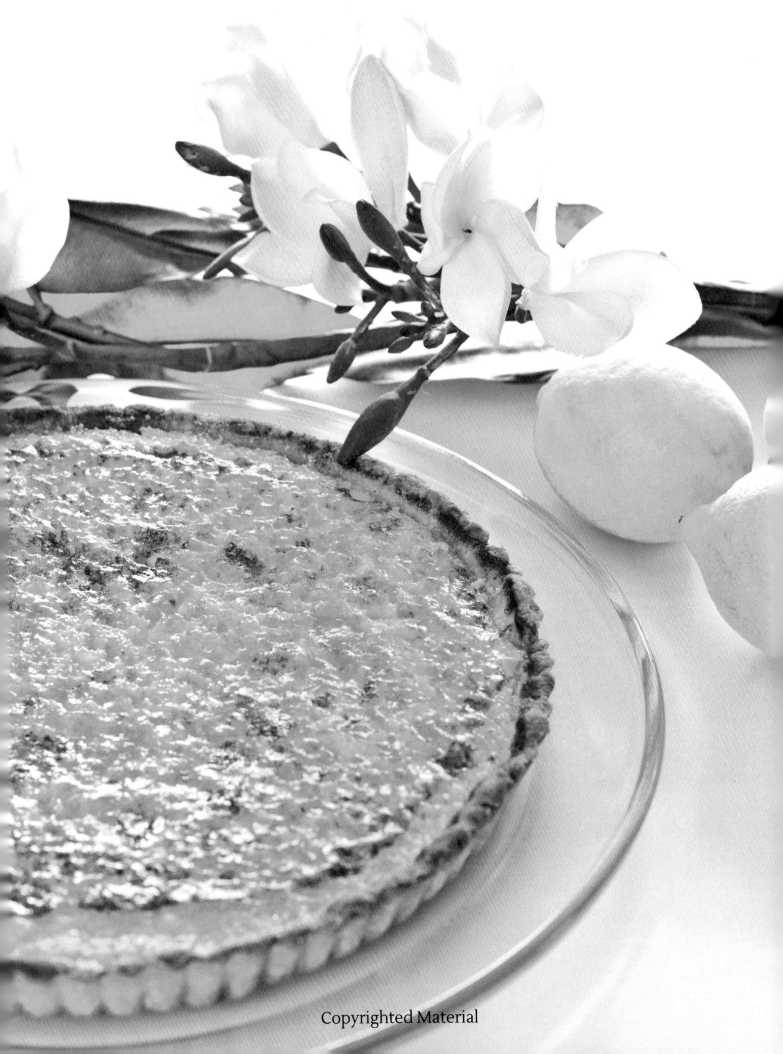

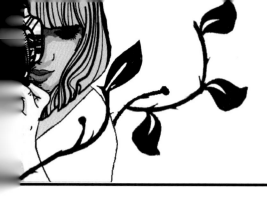

Lemon Tart

For the pastry:

100gms/4.7oz white rice flour

33gms/1.16oz brown rice flour

22gms/0.8oz tapioca flour

45gms/1.6oz potato starch

pinch of salt

1 heaped tbsp sugar

100gms/3.5oz butter

1 medium egg

For the filling:

150gms/5.4oz butter, melted

1/2 cup lemon juice

grated rind of 2 lemons

5 eggs

1/2 cup castor sugar

For the pastry:

1. Blend all the dry ingredients in a food processor.

2. Add the butter cut into small pieces to the food processor and process until fine crumbs form.

3. Add the egg and process until it forms a dough.

4. Remove from the processor and add a little more rice flour if it is too wet – this depends on the size of your egg.

5. Press into a greased tart dish with a removable bottom and place in the fridge for 30 minutes.

6. Preheat the oven to 180°C/360°F.

7. Place baking paper in the base of the tart and fill with rice or dried beans and blind bake for 20 minutes.

For the filling:

8. Beat all the ingredients together.

9. Pour into the prepared pastry shell.

10. Place in the oven and bake for 25 minutes or until set.

11. Cool in the baking tin and then remove.

Strands of My Life

VEGETARIAN DINNER

Potato rosti pizza

A crunchy quinoa salad

Chocolate banana tarts

Serves 6

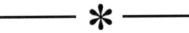

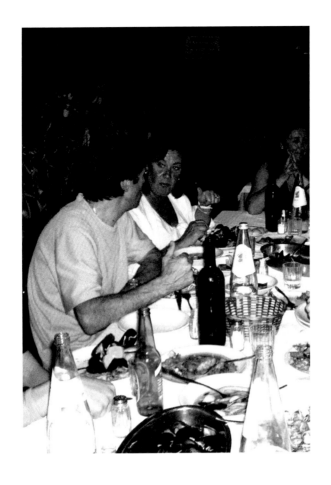

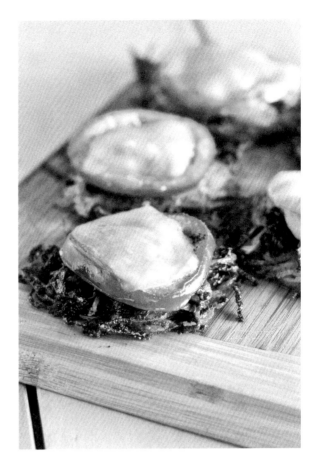

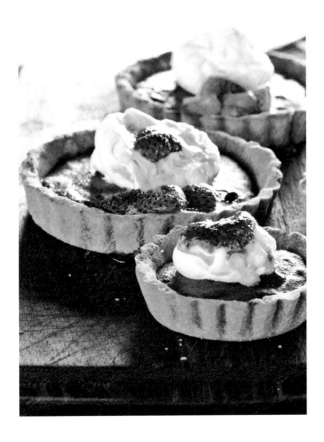

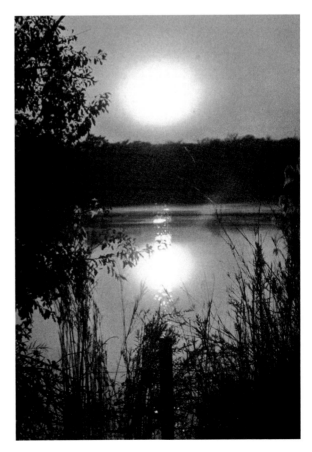

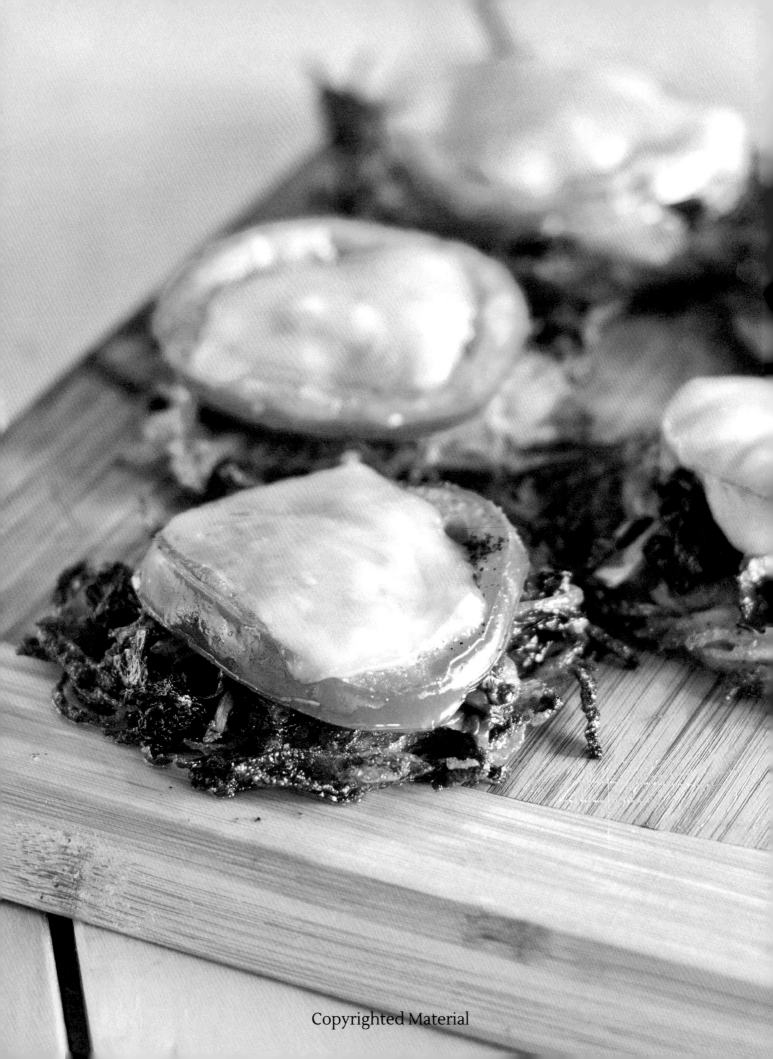

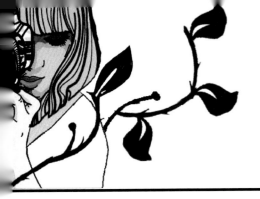

Potato Rosti Pizzas

4 potatoes, peeled

Salt & pepper

A bag of spinach

1 tomato

Hard cheese or mozzarella

Coconut oil & butter

1. Preheat the oven to 180°C/350°F.
2. Grate the potatoes in a food processor or with a hand grater.
3. Squeeze out all the water and dry with a clean tea towel.
4. Season with salt and pepper and mix well.
5. Melt the butter and coconut oil in a frying pan.
6. Place heaped spoonfuls of the mixture into the hot oil/butter mixture and shape into rough, flat circles.
7. Fry until golden on both sides.
8. Meanwhile wilt the spinach in another frying pan with a little butter. Season with salt and pepper.
9. Place the cooked rosti on baking paper on a baking tray.
10. Place a layer of spinach on top of each one.
11. Follow with a slice of tomato and season.
12. Layer a slice of cheese on top and place the tray in the oven for about 5 mins until the cheese is melted.

Strands of My Life

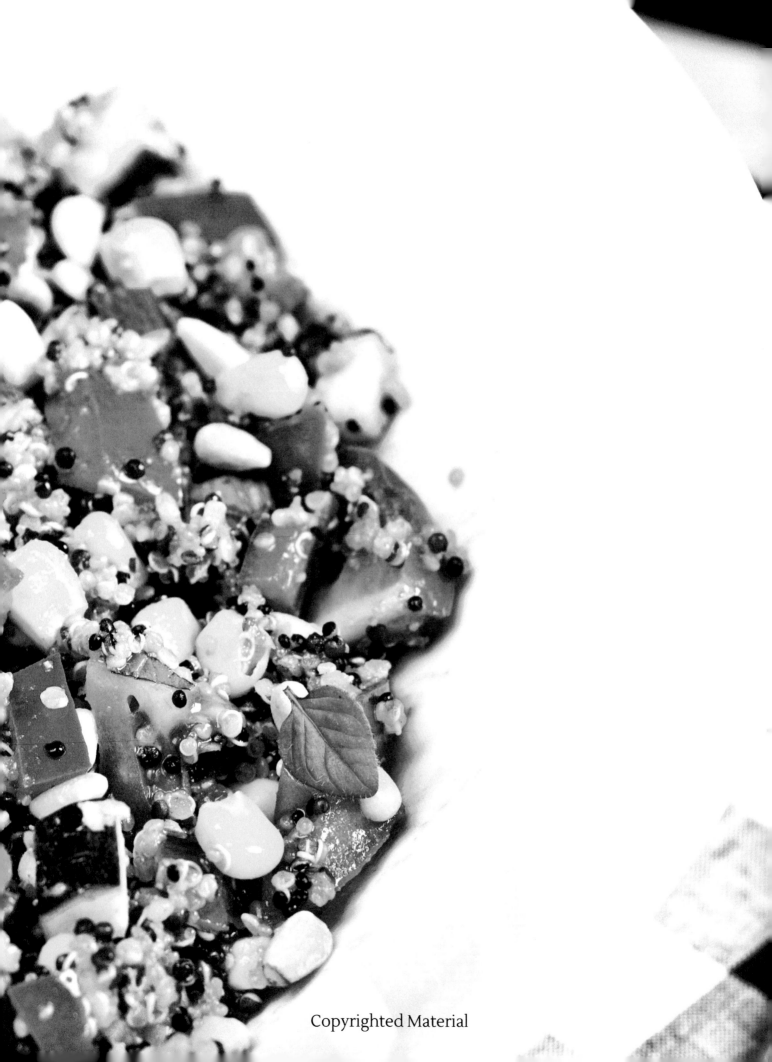

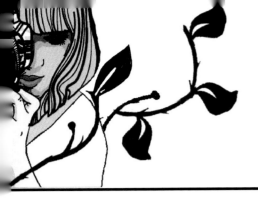

Crunchy Quinoa Salad

Quinoa

Corn (freshly cooked and cut off the cob)

Zucchini

Leeks (green part only)

Fresh oregano

Tomatoes

Red bell pepper

Pine nuts

Vinaigrette dressing

1. Cook the quinoa according to the instructions on the packet.

2. Cool completely.

3. Chop up the vegetables into small chunks.

4. Chop the oregano finely.

5. Toast the pine nuts.

6. Mix everything together.

7. Dress with a vinaigrette made with olive oil, balsamic vinegar, salt and pepper.

8. This salad will keep fresh in the fridge for a few days.

Note: 1/2 cob of corn is low Fodmap

Strands of My Life

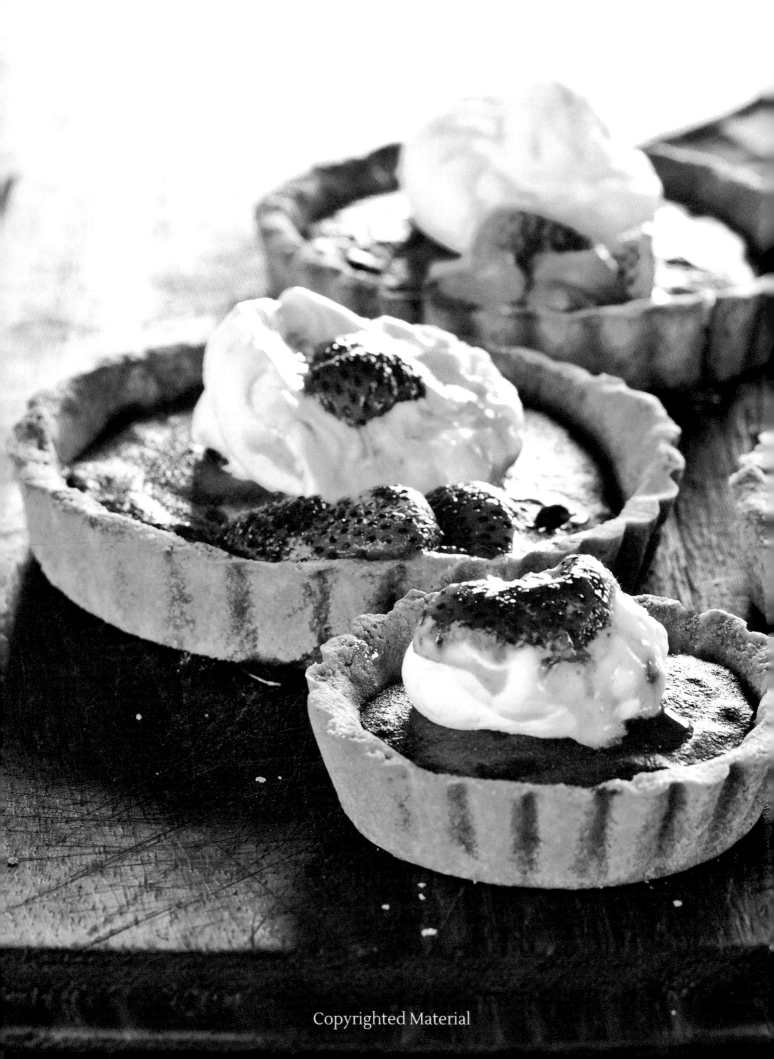

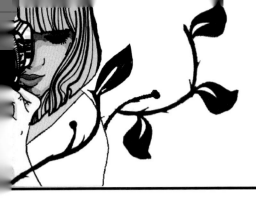

Chocolate Banana Tarts

For the pastry:

100gms/4.7oz white rice flour

33gms/1.16oz brown rice flour

22gms/0.8oz tapioca flour

45gms/1.6oz potato starch

pinch of salt

1 heaped tbsp sugar

100gms/3.5oz butter

1 medium egg

For the filling:

3 bananas

1 tbsp maple syrup

1/4 cup coconut oil

1/3 cup cocoa

For the pastry:

1. Blend all the dry ingredients in a food processor.
2. Add the butter cut into small pieces to the food processor and process until fine crumbs form.
3. Add the egg and process until it forms a dough.
4. Remove from the processor and add a little more rice flour if it is too wet – this depends on the size of your egg.
5. Press into greased tart dishes with removable bottoms and place in the fridge for 30 minutes.
6. Preheat the oven to 180°C/350°F.
7. Place baking paper in the base of the tart and fill with rice or dried beans and blind bake for 20 minutes.

For the filling:

8. Melt the coconut oil if it is solid.
9. Place everything in a food processor and process until smooth.
10. Spoon into the cooked and cooled pastry shells.
11. Refrigerate until cold.
12. Serve with cream and a few stewed strawberries.

(Note: eat only a small tart at a sitting.)

Strands of My Life

LOVERS' DINNER DATE

Pesto polenta tapas

Tapioca cheese bread rolls

Thai-style chicken salad

Blueberry mousse dessert

Serves 2

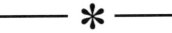

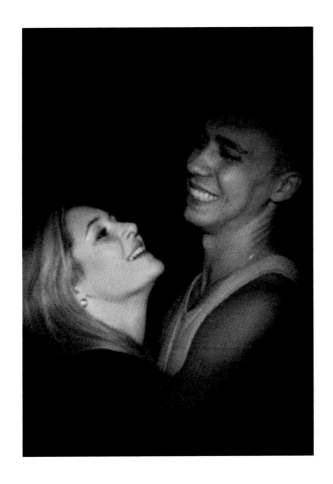

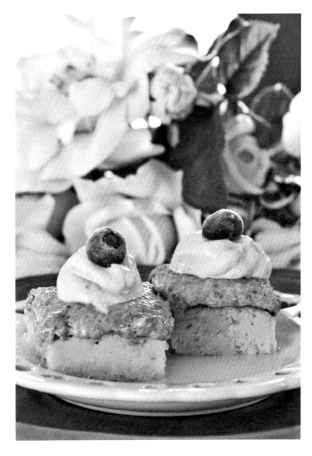

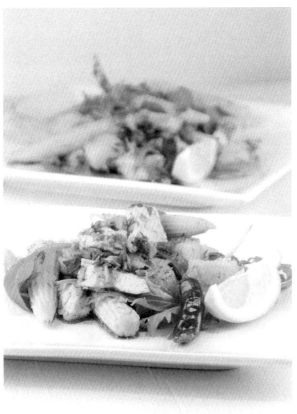

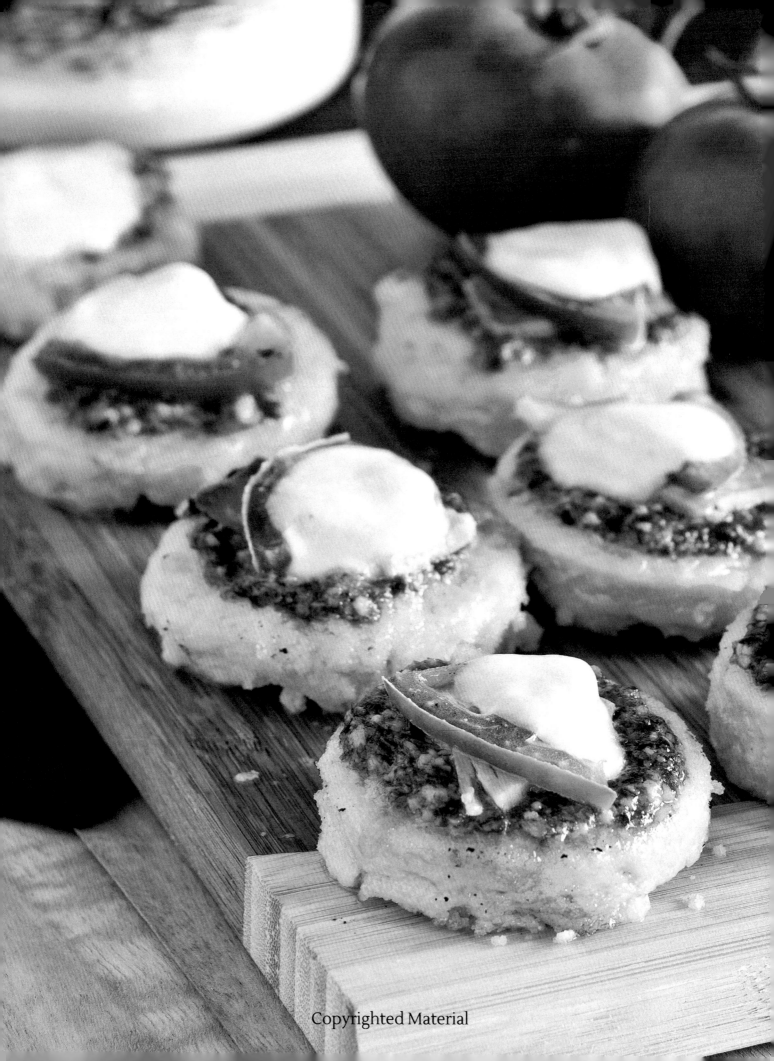

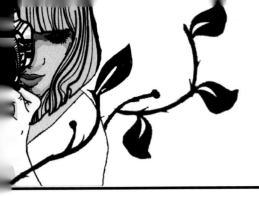

Pesto, Mozzarella Polenta Appetizers

For the pesto:

A bunch of basil

2 tbsp pine nuts

40gms/1.4oz Parmesan

1 tbsp garlic-infused oil

1/2 cup olive oil

Salt & pepper

For the polenta:

1 liter /2.1 pints water

250gms/8.8oz polenta

To assemble:

1 big slice of ham

Several small bocconcini

(mozzarella balls)

2 tomatoes

For the pesto:

1. Place everything except the oils in a food processor and process until well chopped.

2. Drizzle in the combined oils while the machine is running.

For the polenta:

3. Cook the polenta according to the instructions on the packet.

4. Remove and immediately pour onto a big chopping board.

5. Smooth it out as much as possible to an even thickness – about ¾"/2cm.

6. Using a small glass, cut out rounds and oil them lightly.

7. Put them onto a hot grill and leave until grill marks appear. You can do both sides but one is enough.

To assemble:

8. With grilled sides facing up, slather on a little pesto and top with a small piece of ham, a ¼ of a slice of tomato and ½ a tiny bocconcini mozzarella.

9. Place under the grill for about 5 minutes

Strands of My Life

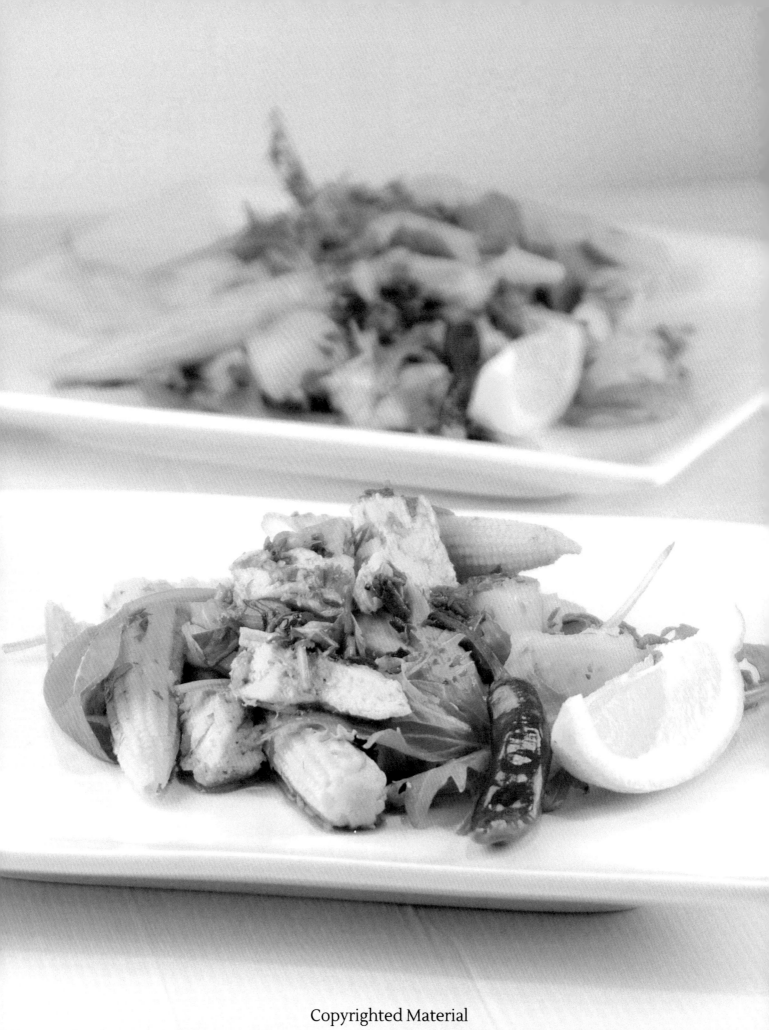

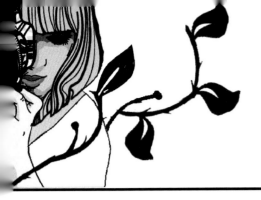

Thai-Style Chicken Salad

For the salad:

300g/10.5oz new potatoes, chopped up

A can of baby corn

2 spring onions (green part) sliced

2 cooked chicken breasts, sliced

1 tbsp chopped coriander

Salt & pepper

Wedges of lemon as a garnish

For the dressing:

3 tbsp of sesame oil

1 tbsp lemon juice

1/2 tbsp soy sauce

1 tbsp chopped coriander

1 chilli, deseeded and finely sliced

For the salad:

1. Boil the potatoes until tender, drain and cool.

2. Cook the chicken breasts in a pan with a little olive oil, then slice up.

3. Combine all the ingredients in a large bowl.

For the dressing:

4. Mix the dressing ingredients well and pour over the salad.

5. Garnish with the lemon wedges and a few extra coriander leaves.

Note: 1/2 cob of corn is low Fodmap

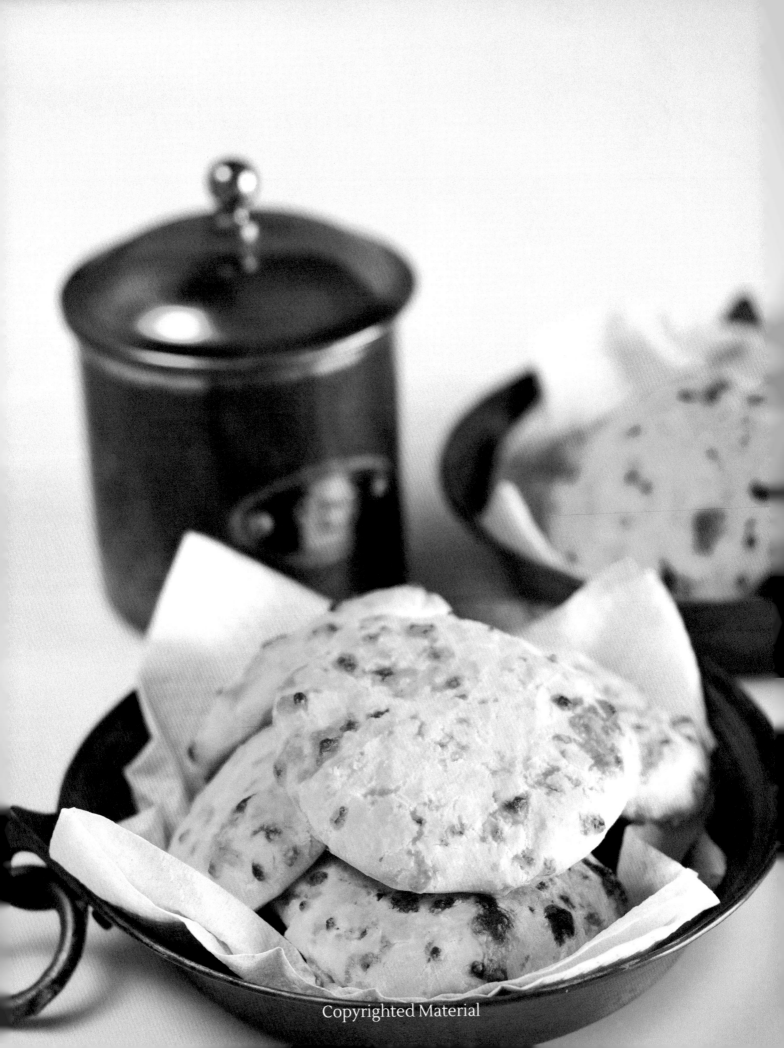

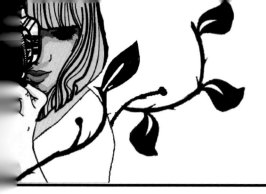

Tapioca Cheese Bread Rolls

2.5 cups tapioca flour

3 cups mozzarella cheese

1 tsp baking powder

Pinch of salt

113gms/4oz butter

2 large eggs

1-2 tbsp water, if needed

1. Preheat oven to 350°F/180°C.

2. Mix the flour, cheese, baking powder and salt in a food processor.

3. Add the softened butter and eggs and blend until it clumps together.

4. Add a little water if necessary.

5. Make small rounds of the dough and place on baking paper on an oven tray.

6. Bake for about 10 minutes until cooked.

7. Serve while warm.

Strands of My Life

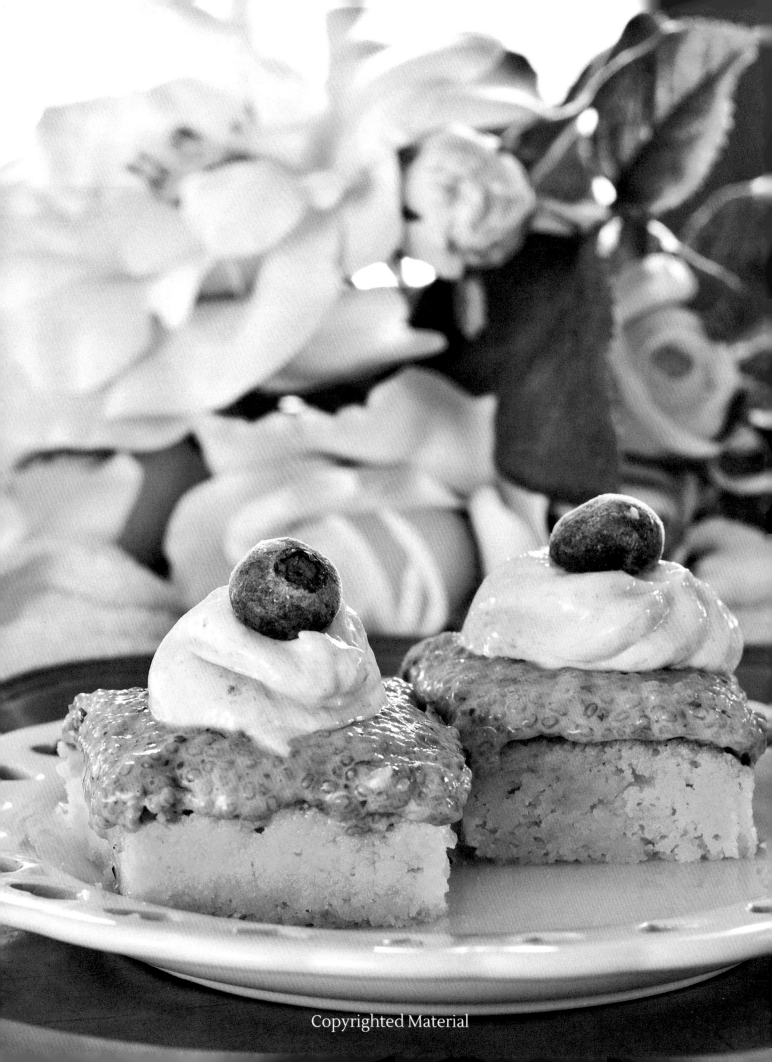

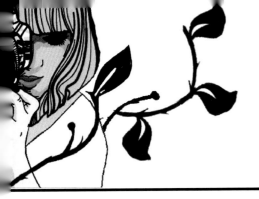

Blueberry Mousse Dessert

For the cake:

200gms/7oz softened butter

150gms/5.5oz caster sugar

4 eggs

110gms/3.9oz white rice flour

30gms/1oz potato starch

30gms/1oz tapioca flour

250gms/8.8oz mashed potato

2 tsp baking powder

For the mousse:

2 cups coconut cream

1/2 cup blueberries (fresh or frozen)

3 tbsp maple syrup

1/2 cup chia seeds

1 tsp gelatin (dissolved in 1 tbsp hot water)

For the topping:

250gms/8.8ozs cream cheese

1 tbsp icing sugar

1 ripe banana

Note: see page 19 for dairy alternatives

For the cake:

1. Preheat the oven to 180°C/350°F.
2. Butter and line a 20cm cake tin.
3. Beat the sugar and butter together until light and fluffy then add the eggs one at a time while still beating.
4. Sift the flours and baking powder together and add to the wet ingredients.
5. Add the mashed potato and mix through.
6. Pour into the tin and bake for 35-40 minutes or until a skewer comes out clean.
7. Cool a little then tip out onto a wire rack.
8. Cool completely before piling on the topping.

For the mousse:

9. Place everything in a food processor and process until combined.
10. Pour on top of the cooled cake.
11. Place in the fridge until completely set.
12. Cut into squares.

For the topping:

13. Place all ingredients into a food processor and process until smooth.
14. Pipe a little on top of each square.
15. Keep in the fridge.
16. Top each with a blueberry.

Strands of My Life

MIDNIGHT FEAST

Creamy fusilli salad

Beef open sandwiches

Oatmeal whoopie pies

Serves 6

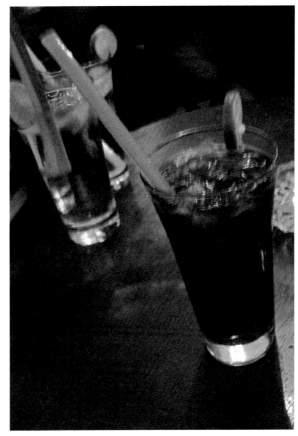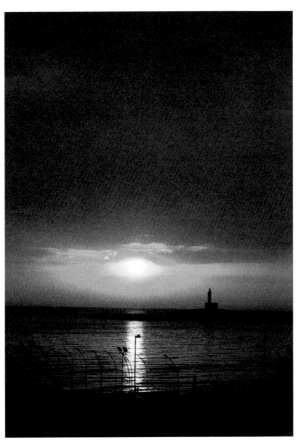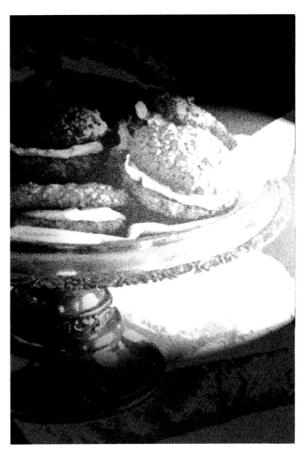

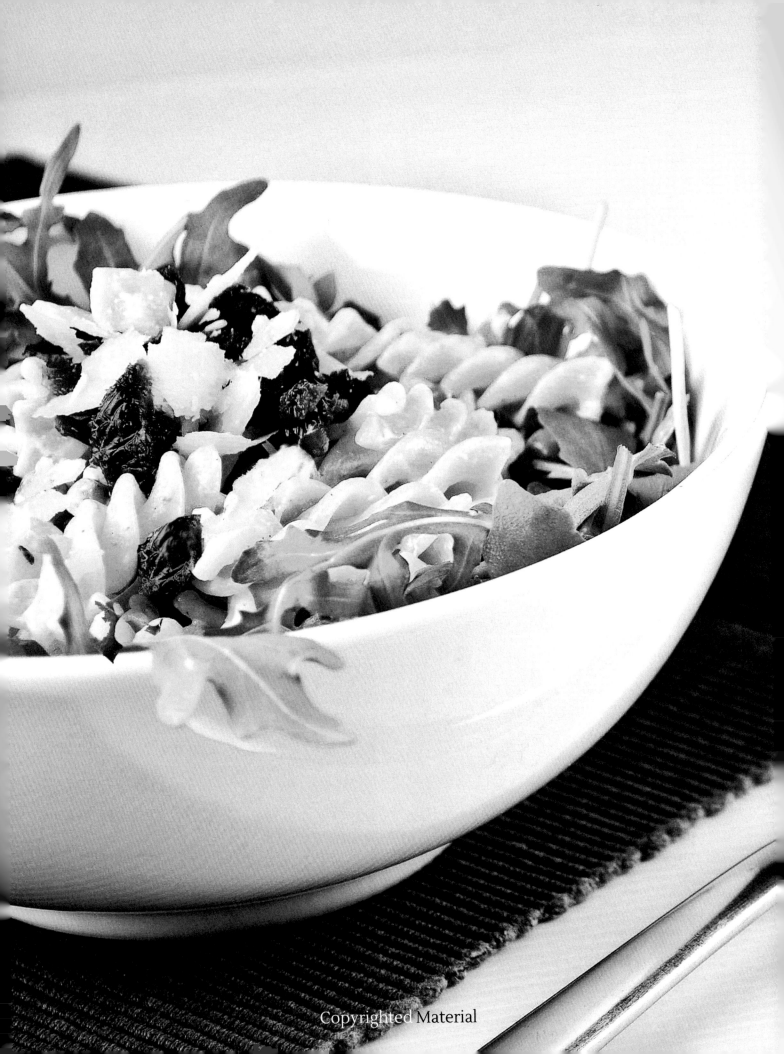

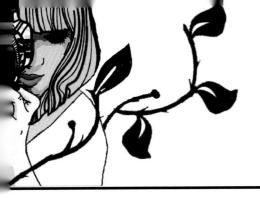

Creamy Fusilli Salad

Juice of 1/2 a lemon

Zest of 1 lemon

125g/4.4oz sour cream

3 tbsp milk

Tabasco sauce

Salt and black pepper

500gms/17.6oz fusilli pasta

1 packet of arugula

10 sundried tomatoes, sliced

Shaved parmesan

Note: see page 19 for dairy alternatives

1. Boil the pasta as usual.

2. Mix together the first six ingredients to create the sauce.

3. Drain pasta and add the sauce and all but a few sundried tomatoes.

4. Dress the plates with the arugula and place the pasta in the middle and decorate with the rest of the sundried tomatoes and scatter over the parmesan.

Strands of My Life

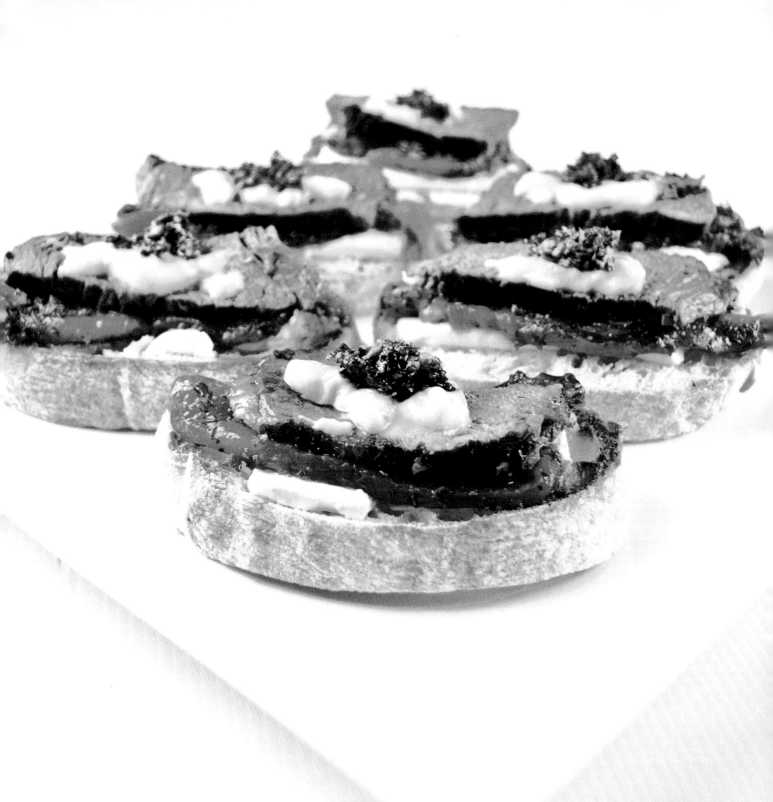

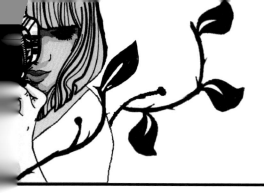

Beef and Roasted Pepper Bruschetta

A thick slab of sirloin steak

Feta cheese

2 red peppers

Parsley

Coriander

Garlic -infused olive oil

Pepper & salt

Gluten-free bread – sliced (page 75)

Horseradish sauce

Home-made pesto (page 49)

1. Grill the steak until medium rare and let rest for 5 minutes. Cut into slices.

2. Char the peppers under the grill in the oven or on the grill on the stove top until the skin is black. Remove the skins.

3. Slice up the peppers and mix with a few tablespoons of garlic oil, chopped up parsley and coriander. Season the mixture.

4. Toast one side of the sliced bread, then remove and place a slice of feta on top. Place under the grill again for a short time.

5. Top with the peppers and a slice or two of steak.

6. Place a small teaspoon of horseradish in the middle of the steak and top with a blob of pesto.

Strands of My Life

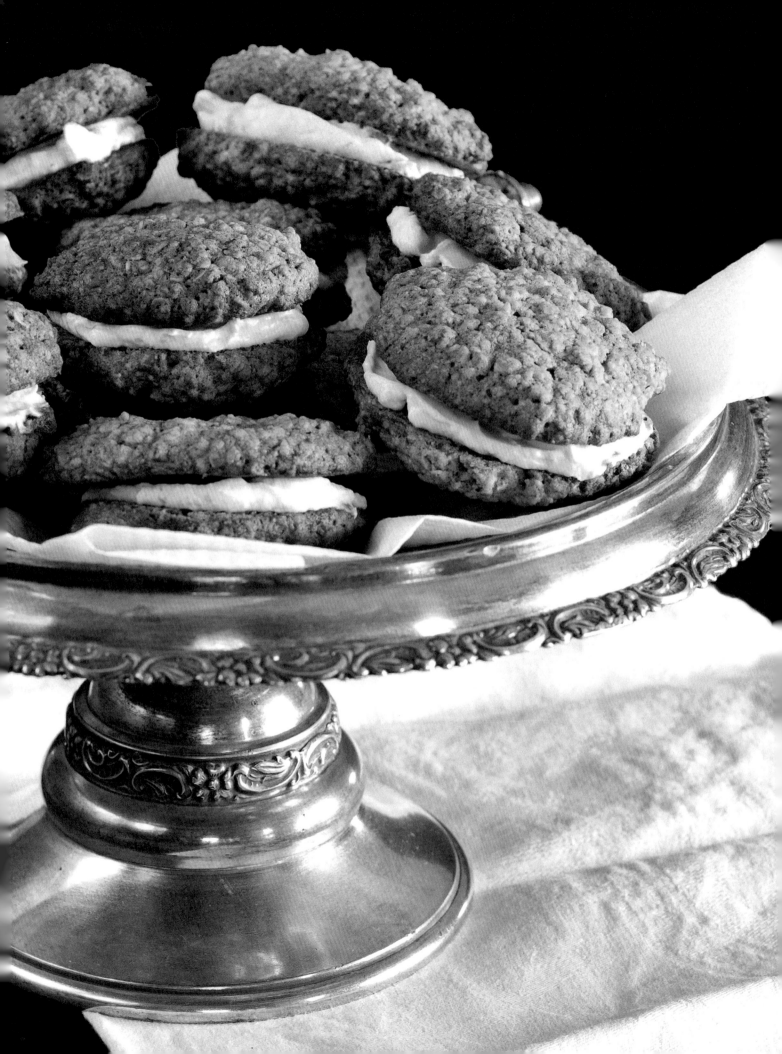

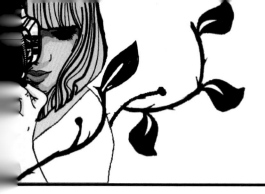

Oatmeal Whoopie Pies

For The whoopies:

170gms/6oz soft butter

2/3 cup brown sugar

1 egg

1 tsp vanilla

1/4 cup white rice flour

1/4 cup tapioca flour

1/4 cup potato starch

1/2 tsp baking soda

1 tsp xantham gum

1/2 tsp salt

1/2 tsp cinnamon

2.5 cups of rolled oats

For the filling:

100gms/3.5oz cream cheese

1 soft banana

2 tbsp icing sugar

1. Preheat oven to 180°C/350°F.

2. Line a baking tray with baking paper.

3. Cream the butter and sugar until light and fluffy.

4. Add the egg and vanilla and beat some more.

5. Sift the dry ingredients, except the oats, together.

6. Add the flours to the butter mixture.

7. Add the oats and mix well.

8. Spoon spoonfuls of the mixture onto the baking paper and mound into small domes. Leave a space between because they will spread a little.

9. Bake for 8-10 minutes.

10. Cool a while to firm up and then remove from the tray to a cooling rack.

11. Place the banana, icing sugar and cream cheese in a food processor and process until smooth or mash the banana and beat into the cream cheese and sugar with a wooden spoon.

12. Spread the cream cheese over half the cookies and top with the other halves.

13. Keep in the fridge.

Note: see page 19 for dairy alternatives

Strands of My Life

INDEX

Dinner with Friends

Formal Dinner Party

Family Dinner

Vegetarian Dinner

Lovers' Dinner Date

Midnight Feast

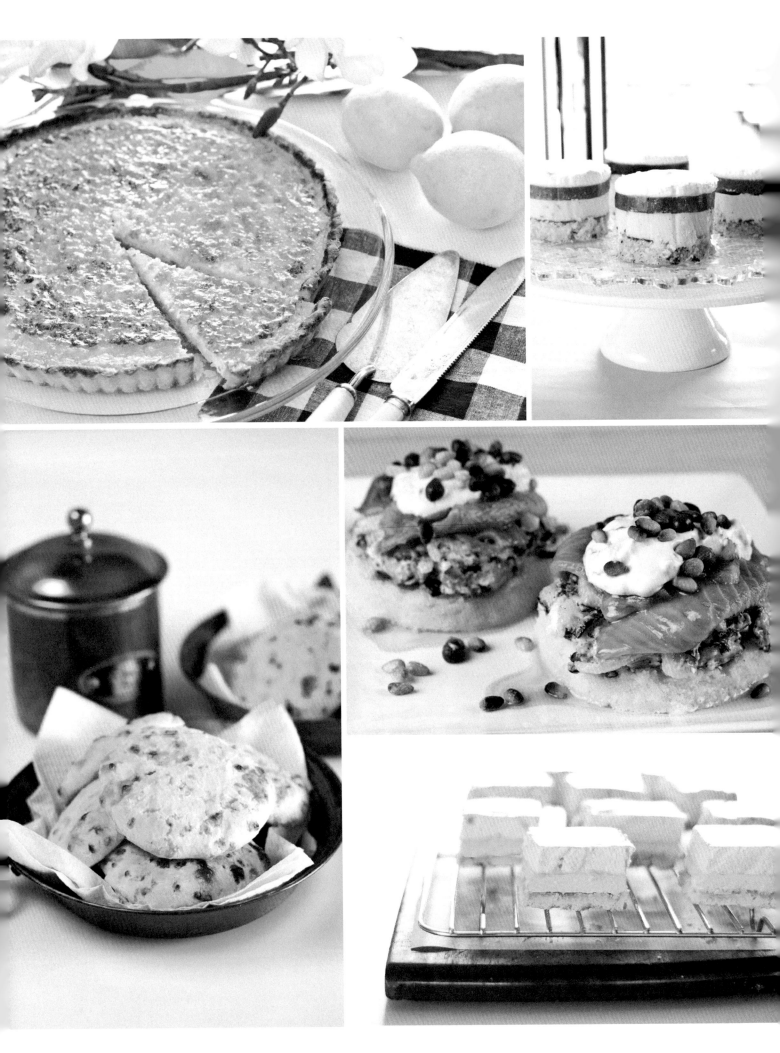

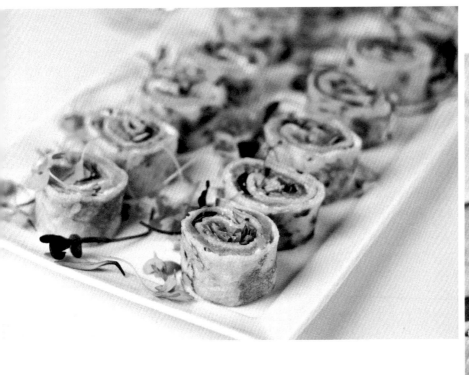
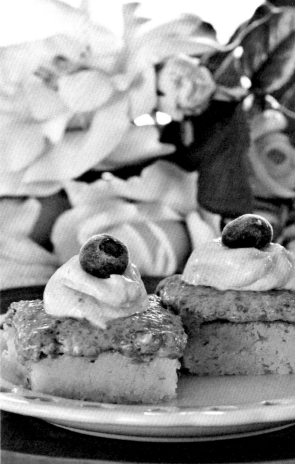
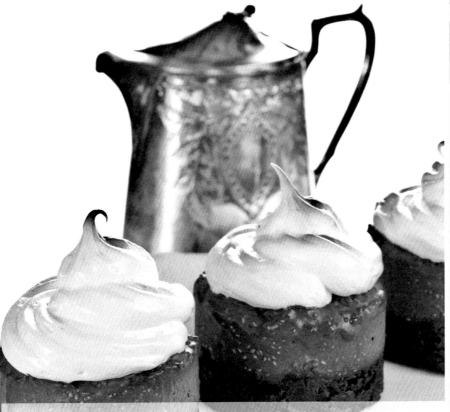
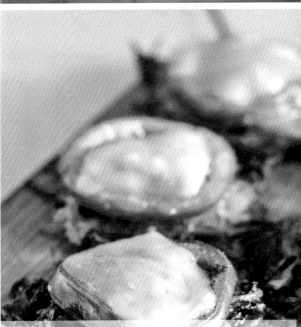

For more information on Suzanne Perazzini and her recipes, visit her food blog: www.strandsofmylife.com
If you would like to join her low Fodmap diet program, fill in the form on this page: www.strandsofmylife.com/inspiredlife
If you have enjoyed this book, please leave a review on Amazon: http://amzn.to/1r2N36f

Made in the USA
San Bernardino, CA
29 December 2017